FOOT SOLDIERS

Armed with Love

Heartbeat International's First Forty Years

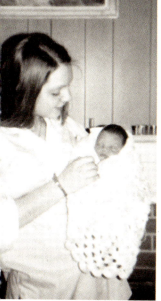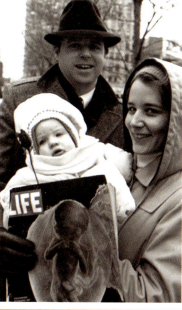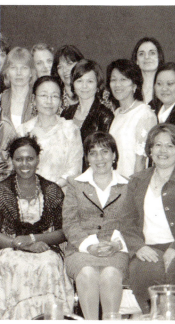

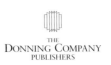

THE
DONNING COMPANY
PUBLISHERS

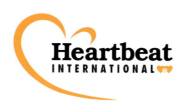

FOOT SOLDIERS

Armed with Love

Heartbeat International's First Forty Years

Margaret H. (Peggy) Hartshorn, Ph.D.

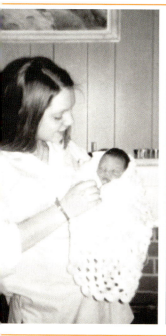
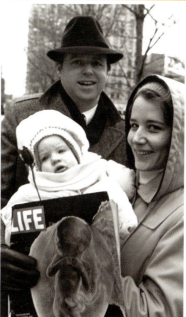
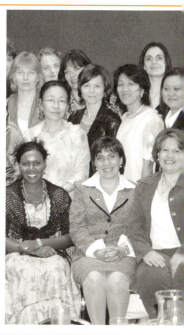

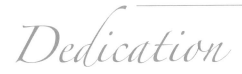

Dedication

This history is dedicated to the early visionaries and founders of
Heartbeat International, especially to Sister Paula Vandegaer, the late
Dr. John Hillabrand, Lore Maier, and to the hundreds of thousands of
foot soldiers, armed with love, who have followed in their steps these
first forty years.

Margaret H. Hartshorn

Copyright © 2011 by Heartbeat International

All rights reserved, including the right to reproduce this work in any form whatsoever without permission in writing
from the publisher, except for brief passages in connection with a review. For information, please write:

The Donning Company Publishers
184 Business Park Drive, Suite 206
Virginia Beach, VA 23462

Steve Mull, General Manager
Barbara Buchanan, Office Manager
Pamela Koch, Senior Editor
Chad H. Casey, Graphic Designer
Priscilla Odango, Imaging Artist
Jeanie Akins, Project Research Coordinator
Tonya Washam, Marketing Specialist
Pamela Engelhard, Marketing Advisor

Ed Williams, Project Director

Library of Congress Cataloging-in-Publication Data

Hartshorn, Margaret H., 1947-
  Foot soldiers armed with love : Heartbeat International's first forty years / Margaret H. (Peggy) Hartshorn.
    p. cm.
  ISBN 978-1-57864-721-7 (soft cover : alk. paper)
  1. Heartbeat International. 2. Abortion—Religious aspects—Christianity. 3. Pregnant women—Services for. 4.
Pro-life movement. I. Title.
  HQ767.25.H37 2011
  363.460973—dc23

                    2011039061

Printed in the United States of America at Walsworth Publishing Company

Table of Contents

Foreword

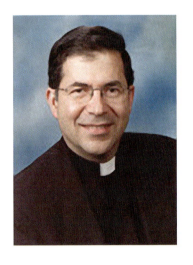

All of us at Priests for Life are convinced that the progress of the pro-life movement rests upon our ability to show our culture that we do not point fingers of condemnation but, rather, extend hands of mercy to lift up from despair those who might abort or who have aborted their children. These sisters and brothers of ours do not act out of "freedom of choice," but out of the feeling of having no freedom and no choice. Heartbeat International, and all its affiliate centers, change that completely, as this fascinating forty-year history demonstrates. By saving lives and healing wounds, they reveal the true face of the pro-life movement and, ultimately, the Face of God Himself. The children for whom we advocate, their moms and dads, and those who help them, all have something in common: *a heartbeat.* May the work of Heartbeat International continue to show the solidarity that God intends us all to experience, as the Culture of Life increasingly dominates and replaces the culture of death.

Fr. Frank Pavone
National Director
Priests for Life

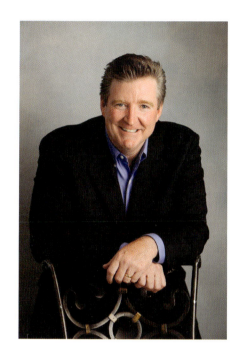

As this history lovingly documents, from humble beginnings, Heartbeat International has grown to become one of the most significant and far-reaching pregnancy help ministries in the world. The numbers speak for themselves: about 1,200 pregnancy help ministries in 50 countries; 700,000 clients served every year by a network of more than 25,000 volunteers; and most significantly, an average of 2,000 babies saved *every week* by the Heartbeat network. But it's not about the numbers, is it? Behind the figures and statistics lie individual souls, each carrying the fingerprints of their Creator. Whether it's an expectant mom considering whether or not to terminate her pregnancy, a grieving woman agonizing over her tragic choice, or a tiny, helpless baby growing in the womb with no one to defend her, Heartbeat is involved in the active, day-to-day mission of touching individual lives with God's grace. I can't imagine a more important calling than that! May the Lord continue to bless all Heartbeat does, expand its influence, and use Heartbeat to defend the defenseless and advance the pro-life cause for years to come.

Jim Daly
President
Focus on the Family

Acknowledgments

The information and stories contained in this history of Heartbeat International's first forty years have been gathered with a great deal of help from two sources: Heartbeat's files and records, and some of the people who experienced our history first hand.

For the years when we were known as AAI, Alternatives to Abortion International, I have information from all three of our founders: Sister Paula Vandegaer, the late Dr. John Hillabrand, and Lore Maier.

Sister Paula Vandegaer, the original secretary of the AAI Board and director of the West Coast Office of AAI in Los Angeles from 1977 to 1986, allowed me to search her files in Los Angeles for information on AAI's early history, she sent pictures, and she provided me two extensive in-person interviews (one of which is captured on video), and several phone calls to check facts.

I am indebted to the late Lore Maier, our first executive director, who kept the originals of AAI minutes, correspondence, and publications in Toledo, Ohio, even after the corporate office was moved to New York in the 1980s. Copies of these documents that she sent to New York were later destroyed in a fire. Lore handed her precious originals to me, in person, when I became president of Heartbeat International.

Dr. John Hillabrand's nurse, Esther Applegate, who was also an original regional consultant for AAI, made a special trip to Columbus from her retirement home in Longmont, Colorado, to provide us with an interview and share her memories of Dr. Hillabrand and the early years of AAI. Raena Avalon, one of the early clients of Dr. John and Lore, also gave me extensive interviews and allowed us to videotape her memories.

Alice Brown, one of the first presidents (chairman of the board) of AAI, also shared information with us, especially her conjecture on the original "seeds" for AAI. She and her husband, Dr. Frank Brown, were part of a group that preceded AAI, and that brought together many of those who later were involved in that founding and the founding of several other pro-life organizations. It was a group who regularly attended annual, weeklong "Family Life Seminars" on the campus of St. John's University at Collegeville, Minnesota, in the mid-1960s and early 1970s, organized by Father Paul Marx, professor of sociology at St. John's University (who later founded Human Life International). According to Alice, "Each year he was able to attract an internationally prominent faculty representing the various disciplines of medicine, psychology, theology, social work, law, philosophy, and others. Dr. John Hillabrand and Lore Maier were among the large number of regular attendees, from across the United States and beyond. . . . It seems to us that it was in this environment of sharing [that] Dr. John and Lore came to recognize the need and desirability of a means for ongoing dialogue, communication, and education and thus the concept of AAI." This does seem accurate since the first AAI Academy (now called the Heartbeat International Annual Conference) was held on the campus of St. John's University in 1972.

For facts on the history of Heartbeat International from 1993 to the present, I am indebted to the current Heartbeat staff, who have spent many hours in sorting and compiling information from our written and pictorial files, jogging my memory, and "fact checking." I thank particularly Kathy Chellis, Virginia Cline, Debbie Schirtzinger, Betty McDowell, and Jor-El Godsey. For invaluable help with the pictures and manuscript, I thank Lauren Chenoweth and Christy Poloni. For insightful comments on the early drafts of the text, I thank Heartbeat International Board member Chris Dattilo, Heartbeat Ministry Service Vice President Jor-El Godsey, and my husband Mike, who has been my mainstay and most faithful Heartbeat supporter throughout the years covered by this history.

Finally, most of the stories contained in this history come from my own memory, faulty as it is sometimes! I have tried to represent our history as accurately as possible, but I am ultimately responsible for any inaccuracies in this story of Heartbeat International's remarkable first forty years.

My Story as a Foot Soldier

It was seemingly just another cold winter day in Columbus, Ohio. I had left our apartment and was driving north on High Street, the major north/south artery toward The Ohio State University where I was working on a graduate degree. It was January 22, 1973. My mind was on a meeting with my academic advisor, but I had the car radio on, vaguely listening to a program on National Public Radio. Then the newscaster made an announcement that stunned me. The Supreme Court of the United States, ruling in a case called *Roe v. Wade*, had declared unconstitutional every one of the existing state laws that restricted abortion: a woman now had a "right to privacy" that covered a decision to have an abortion at any time during her pregnancy. In one fell swoop, the Supreme Court had declared unconstitutional every state law in our country that protected unborn children and their mothers from abortion! At first, I could not believe my ears. As soon as I saw my husband (an attorney in his first year of practice), I thought, he could go to the law library and get a copy of the decision. Surely, the radio had it wrong!

My mind raced back to my college years in California, the state that was among the four states to first liberalize their abortion laws in 1967. The ethics professor at our Catholic women's college warned our class in 1968, "Mark my words, in five years abortion will be legal all over the United States." I remembered a soft gasp of surprise and denial coming from the class at that time. Had that horrible prophecy come true? And had I not noticed what had been happening, preoccupied as I was with graduate school, my young marriage, the death of my father—all of which seemed to be the most important events in the world at that time?

If this news was correct, I knew I had to do something. For me, this was a never-to-be-forgotten day, seared into memory, like other days in history when the United States suffered surprise attacks, December 7, 1941 (Pearl Harbor Day), or September 11, 2001 (the crumbling of the World Trade Center). For me, it was as dramatic a moment as when St. Paul got knocked off his horse.

▶ *Peggy and Mike Hartshorn with their daughter Katy, January 22, 1980, at the State House in Columbus, Ohio, for the annual commemoration of the Supreme Court decision* Roe v. Wade. *Mike holds* LIFE *magazine, featuring the famous photos of life in the womb, taken by photographer Lennart Nilsson. This magazine was one of the best educational materials used in the pro-life movement at that time. The goal of the movement was to convince the public that human life began at conception, a fact that the Supreme Court had said was unsettled.*

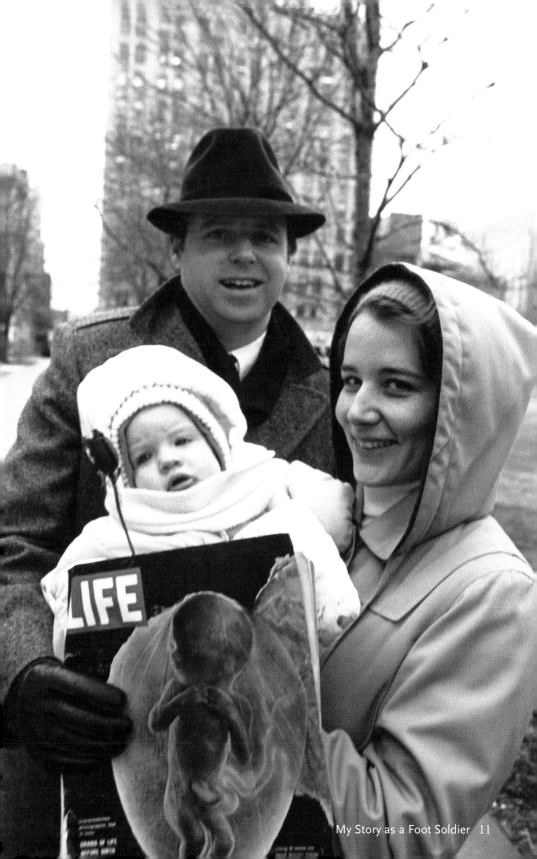

I didn't fully realize then how that day would change my life, nor how God was already preparing me, and thousands of others, to become foot soldiers for Him in the battle for the sanctity of every person's life. I did not know then that I would be in the battle most of my life, and that the battle was ultimately the battle of good vs. evil. Nor did I know that the "army for life" that I would be joining, along with my husband, had been in formation well before January 22, 1973.

Raised in a small town in Ohio, in a devout family with Catholic priests and nuns on my father's side and Protestant missionaries, church organists, and choir members on my mother's side, I went to college in the San Francisco Bay area in the mid-1960s. I saw, with amazement, billboards advertising abortion clinics being put up in 1967, after California legalized abortion. I had been shocked when our ethics professor predicted that abortion would become legal throughout our country.

But that was San Francisco, at the same place and time that the hippies were roaming the streets, experimenting with drugs, and singing, "Make love, not war." And on the nearby campus of the University of California at Berkeley, anti-Vietnam War demonstrators were burning down buildings. During the same years, we witnessed the assassinations of Martin Luther King Jr. and Bobby Kennedy. The world seemed topsy-turvy.

When I returned to Ohio for marriage to my high school sweetheart Mike, and for graduate school, I was lulled into thinking that the world was being right-sided again. I had no idea that the sexual revolution of the sixties, that I had watched unfolding in San Francisco, was not an aberration but was to become the "new normal" and, in fact, would be taken to extremes I could not then have imagined. This revolution was the culmination of a carefully orchestrated campaign, starting in 1921 with Margaret Sanger and the founding of Planned Parenthood (called the American Birth Control League), to change the sexual mores of the United States and of the world and to control the population (who should be born, to whom, and exactly when and where). In terms of sexual mores, their goal was to make sure that sexual intimacy was separated from a lifetime commitment to marriage, and especially separated from children. Since birth control has an inevitable failure rate, abortion was the "linchpin" of their plan.

Planned Parenthood eventually joined forces with Hugh Hefner and other purveyors of pornography to promote the idea that the purpose of sexual intimacy was solely for pleasure and recreation. They were masters at presenting this idea gradually. They "heated things up" ever so slowly at first so that many in the American public did not even notice it. The early *Playboy* magazines, once hidden behind retail counters, seem almost "innocent" compared to the disgusting pornography ever-present today and readily accessible in our homes through the Internet. College students burning bras in the 1960s seems quaint compared to young children being victimized in sex trafficking and sexual exploitation today. Lesbians holding hands in the 1970s seems somewhat innocent compared to the gay rights parades and the bizarre idea of same sex "marriage" that is proposed as "normal" today.

Some in the generation that grew up in the sixties, and later, have been like the proverbial frog that was oblivious to the fact that the water he was thrown into was intentionally being heated up, ever so gradually. That frog eventually boiled to death. I have always felt extremely blessed that I was like the other frog. Coming from the healthy and normal pond that God designed for me, a strong Christian family that believed in and lived out God's design for life and love, I was thrown into hot water and jumped out.

That's why I reacted with shock and dismay on January 22, 1973. This was a call to action!

I soon found (from the phone book) that Columbus had a Right to Life group. I called and said, "What can I do to help?" The first president of Columbus Right to Life, an economist, Ed O'Boyle, and his wife, pediatrician Meade O'Boyle, took Mike and me under their wing, educating us on the issue and helping us find our place in the young pro-life movement that had actually begun to form during the mid-1960s in response to pro-abortion efforts. At that time, Planned Parenthood and their allies, especially the National Abortion Rights Action League (now NARAL Pro-Choice America), and the Religious Coalition for Abortion Rights were leading the charge to legalize abortion state by state. These groups were also orchestrating just the right case to bring through the court system and eventually before the U.S. Supreme Court, and they found that case in Texas. It was called *Roe v. Wade.*

I became active in right-to-life activities as soon as I could. This coincided with finishing my Ph.D. in English literature and becoming an English and humanities professor at Franklin University in Columbus, Ohio. I also became the volunteer education director of Columbus Right to Life. In addition to showing fetal development and abortion slides to any audience that would watch and listen, I was gathering people together to protest on January 22 each year and demonstrating (with our two adopted infants in a double stroller) in front of abortion clinics as they began to open in Columbus. Actually, we were doing the first "sidewalk counseling" and prayer vigils in front of centers, although we didn't use those terms in those days. Soon I was also testifying in the Ohio legislature in attempts to change the new law of the land, and also working to elect pro-life candidates to office. This is what Columbus Right to Life did. It was the educational, legislative, and political arm and army of the pro-life movement.

Our call to action soon led to a call for even more personal involvement. People were calling the local Right to Life office, needing information for girls with crisis pregnancies, some of whom had been "thrown out" of their homes or been abandoned by boyfriends because they refused to have an abortion. Ed and Meade were housing girls in their home, and they asked if we would be willing to do the same.

When Anne, our first "girl," came to live with us in 1975, little did we know that God was preparing us for a lifetime calling in what was then known as the other arm of the pro-life movement, the service arm, or the "alternatives to abortion" movement. In fact, there existed at that time, unknown to us, a relatively new organization, based in Ohio and founded in 1971, now called Heartbeat International, but then known as AAI, Alternatives to Abortion International. In early 1978, at the first Ohio Right to Life Conference, held in Columbus, Mike and I would meet one of the founders of AAI, Lore Maier, and discover that there was *another* entire army of pro-life warriors that was being raised up by the Lord to provide help and support so that no one would ever feel that abortion was her only alternative.

The discovery of AAI, now Heartbeat International, changed our own lives, in ways we never could have imagined, and the lives of hundreds of thousands of other people who have also discovered this alternate army of foot soldiers, armed not with political action or speeches and debates, but with love. That story is the subject of this book.

On our Marriage Encounter weekend in October of 1978, my husband and I felt called to start a pregnancy help center in Columbus, Ohio, inspired by the work of Lore Maier and that other army of pro-life warriors, plus called to commit to a "couple ministry." Mike and I attended our first AAI Academy (conference) in 1979 and we were "hooked"! We had a hotline installed in our bedroom in late 1980 (to make the phone book deadline for our hotline number), and we opened the doors of our first center, Pregnancy Distress Center, on January 22, 1981. We became foot soldiers armed with love. I thought we would start the center and then go back to Right to Life, but that never happened. I was asked to join the AAI Board at the end of 1986.

One thing would lead to another, as often happens when you say "yes" to the Lord, and I eventually left my position as an English professor at Franklin University (where I had taught full or part time for twenty years) and became the first, full-time, salaried executive director (president) of AAI in 1993. At that time, we also changed our name to Heartbeat International. I have been Heartbeat's president ever since, and I am humbled to be in that position as we come to the end of the first forty years of our history.

There are still 1.2 million abortions performed every year in the United States, and approximately 50 million abortions yearly around the world. But the Heartbeat army is stronger than ever, forty years after its founding, despite direct attacks and every conceivable obstacle that could be thrown in its path. It is armed with and powered by the love of the Lord. What could be more potent?

The story of the founding, struggle for existence, and ultimate advance of the foot soldiers of Heartbeat International will be told in this book. Because I knew personally the founders of Heartbeat, and because my life and the lives of my husband and children have become so intertwined with this extraordinary community of Christian warriors, this history must also be a very <u>personal</u> story. It was impossible for me to write it any other way.

The Army Today and How It Rose Up

If you have picked up this book, chances are that you are already aware of, and perhaps even already a vital part of, the pro-life army of love, raised up by the working of the Holy Spirit and growing exponentially today, that is saving lives—every minute of every day—in a life-changing way. It is tens of thousands of individuals from all expressions of Christianity (Catholic, Protestant, Orthodox, nondenominational), working in a wide variety of pregnancy help ministries, whose vision it is to make abortion unwanted now and unthinkable in future generations. They do this by delivering love, hope, and alternatives in the midst of crisis, one person at a time.

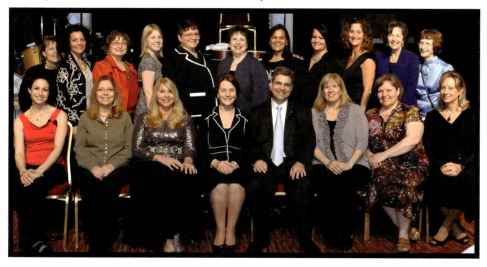

▲ *Staff of Heartbeat International, pictured at our Fortieth Anniversary celebration in Columbus, Ohio, May 20, 2011. Pictured in row one, L to R: Andrea Trudden (Communications and Marketing Director), Debbie Schirtzinger (Affiliation Coordinator), Carla Cole (Executive Vice President), Peggy Hartshorn (President), Jor-El Godsey (Vice President of Ministry Services), Betty McDowell (Director of Affiliate Services), Terri Fox (Development Assistant), Susan Dammann (Medical Clinic Specialist). Row two, L to R: Leslie Malek (Managing Editor), Debra Neybert (Training Specialist), Kathy Chellis (Administrative Assistant), Dawn Lunsford (eLearning Specialist), Robin Mitchell (Bookkeeper), Anita Kremm (Development Manager), Ellen Foell (Legal Counsel), Lauren Chenoweth (Web/Social Media Specialist), Virginia Cline (Public Impact Specialist), Paula Grimsley (Consultant), Bobbie Glotzhober (Director of Operations). Staff not pictured: Christina Poloni (Operations Assistant), Rev. John Ensor (Executive Director for Global Initiatives), Molly Hoepfner (International Coordinator).*

Like the Good Samaritan, they have seen the suffering person abandoned along the way, and they have not passed by. Giving of their own time and treasure, they have gotten involved personally, and are making a lifesaving difference. This life-giving army, with "boots on the ground," right where women are making life or death choices every day, is working in pregnancy help ministries around the world.

The most expansive network of these pro-life pregnancy help ministries, affiliated under one banner, is Heartbeat International. It consists of around 1,200 independent nonprofit groups, in fifty countries, that provide community-based, lifesaving, life-changing, pregnancy-related services, all in the spirit of love and care. In the United States, it was started in the late 1960s, primarily by Catholics (the "first wave" of the pro-life movement), then joined by Evangelicals and other Protestants in the 1980s (the "second wave"), and then enriched especially by African American and Latino Christians, especially in the last fifteen years (the "third wave"). Overseas, it is supported by Catholic, Orthodox, and Protestant Christians—a powerful example of the Body of Christ in this world, being Christ to those in need.

The intention of these Christians is that no woman ever feels forced to have an abortion because of lack of support or practical alternatives. This Heartbeat International army saves lives in a life-changing way. About 2,000 babies and women (and their families) are saved from abortion each week in our network!

The Heartbeat network is supported today almost entirely by private contributions and by about 25,000 volunteers, led by a small number of paid staff and governing boards. So, we are part of one of the greatest volunteer-based movements in history: the pregnancy help movement, sometimes called the alternatives to abortion movement.

Being part of a grassroots and entrepreneurial movement, this army and thus these ministries are diverse. Heartbeat affiliates have a wide selection of services such as crisis pregnancy intervention and support, education and skills training, medical services such as ultrasound to confirm a pregnancy, sexually transmitted disease testing and treatment, limited prenatal care, shelter and housing, adoption, fatherhood programs, abortion recovery, prevention services through abstinence education, and sexual integrity, including fertility appreciation training.

Heartbeat International's central office and leadership (the army headquarters, so to speak!) coordinates this network and links it together. We reach and connect abortion vulnerable women to it through our Option Line (website, toll-free number, and call center), provide leadership training and resources to the army, provide cover and protection from attack (not surprisingly, we have enemies!), and guide and steer this movement as it expands and matures. We try to discern where God is moving, and then lead the army in following Him.

We have been doing this for forty years, a Biblical generation. Our story has parallels to that of the Israelites in the desert for that same period of time: ordinary people who become fearless leaders, doubt and uncertainty, false turns, new directions, enemies, renewed faith, and miraculous

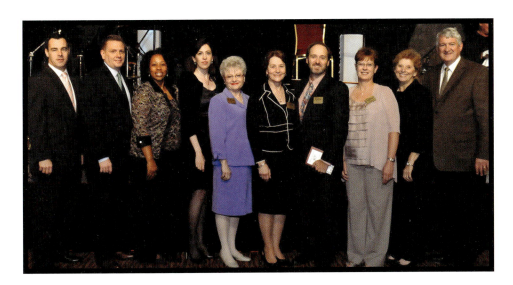

▲ *Governing Board of Heartbeat International, pictured at our Fortieth Anniversary celebration in Columbus, Ohio, May 20, 2011. Pictured, L to R: Brandon McCrary (Insurance One), Thomas Hajdukiewicz (Goldentree Asset Management), Dyxie Lincoln, Pia de Solenni, S.Th.D. (Diatima Consulting, LLC), Julie Parton (Texas Life Connections), Margaret (Peggy) Hartshorn, Ph.D. (President of Heartbeat International), Board Chairman John C. Cissel II (Cornerstone Advisory Services, LLC), Christine Dattilo, Cathy Clark, Ken Clark (Farmer Boys Restaurants). Not pictured: Charles A. Donovan (Susan B. Anthony List), Larry Jacobs (The Howard Center for Family, Religion & Society), Dr. Alveda King (Priests for Life/King for America), Derek A. McCoy (The Maryland Family Alliance and The Maryland Family Council), Dr. Marie Meaney, D.Phil.*

guidance and nourishment from the Lord. Some of the most memorable of these stories will be told in this book.

But we have not reached the "Promised Land!" The bad news is that abortion is still rampant, and the challenges are as great, or greater, than they were forty years ago. But the opportunities are just as great, if not greater.

If Christians want truly to create a Culture of Life, we can learn from, be inspired by, celebrate, and take our "marching orders" from the people and events of Heartbeat's first forty years.

The Foundations

Heartbeat was founded by an ob-gyn physician who was at retirement age, along with a refugee from Nazi Germany and a young Catholic nun who had recently become a licensed social worker. Two were from an aging industrial city on the Great Lakes, Toledo, Ohio, and the other was from the fast-growing city of Los Angeles in the Golden State of California. God used ordinary people, with seemingly extraordinary amounts of foresight, passion, courage, and faith, to begin this

Great Work. This describes our founders and many others who worked alongside them.

Dr. John Hillabrand, Mrs. Lore Maier, and Sister Paula Vandegaer give the founding date of Heartbeat as November 13, 1971, at the first constitutional meeting in Chicago, at the O'Hare Inn, adjacent to O'Hare Airport. Present at the meeting were some of the founders of the approximately sixty help centers and hotlines that were in existence in North America at that time. They saw the need for an affiliation body or an "umbrella group" to help unite and develop this growing movement of pregnancy help and life-giving alternatives to abortion.

While we are called Heartbeat International now, at this meeting we were first named Alternatives to Abortion Incorporated, nicknamed AAI, and so we were called in the first twenty years of our history. Thus, forty years ago, we became the first network of alternatives to abortion services (pregnancy help centers, pregnancy help medical clinics, maternity homes, and adoption agencies) founded in the United States.

But the story of our founding goes back, at least, to the late 1960s. Heartbeat is truly a movement of the Lord, and how do you date the first motions or "trembling" that eventually becomes so strong that it is felt, cannot be ignored, and must even be given a constitution and a name?

The entire pro-life movement started in the 1960s when it became clear that there were forces pushing for legalized abortion in every state, and Heartbeat's story is part of that bigger one. Colorado, California, Oregon, and North Carolina were the first to liberalize their laws in 1967, allowing abortion for "hard cases" such as mental disability of either child or mother, or rape or incest. In 1970, New York allowed abortion on demand up to the twenty-fourth week of pregnancy, and similar laws were passed in Alaska, Hawaii, and the state of Washington. Many people who had never been touched directly by abortion, but who were pro-life and pro-family because of both instinct and deeply held religious beliefs, were abhorred by these developments. Forces organized to counter the efforts to liberalize abortion laws, and they met with great success. Before January 22, 1973, thirty-one states still allowed abortion only to save the life of the mother.

Some people were wise enough to understand completely the well-organized and strategic forces behind the drive to legalize abortion (see introduction). Our founders were among this group. They fully understood the attack on human life and its profound effects on not only individuals but on our entire culture and values underpinning it. They knew that a "safety net" for women and babies was needed.

So they began, in the late 1960s, to develop services such as hotlines and counseling for women in their own communities so that these women would never feel forced into abortion because they thought they had no other alternative. Louise Summerhill founded the first freestanding pregnancy center, called Birthright, in 1968, in Toronto, Canada. The first actual hotline that can be identified in North America was founded in 1971 in Los Angeles, California, and called Lifeline (as part of the Right to Life League of Southern California).

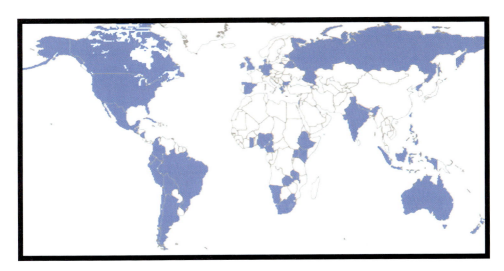

▲ *One-third of the world's countries (shaded) have pregnancy help ministries affiliated with Heartbeat International. We are the most expansive network of life-affirming pregnancy help in the world, and the first network of help ministries founded in the United States, in 1971.*

Some of the pioneers knew each other, but most were generally unaware of the existence of the others until they met in Washington, D.C., in early 1971. (Remember, this was before the Internet!) Monsignor James McHugh, a priest who headed the Family Life department of the United States Conference of Catholic Bishops and who had an overview of what was happening, called a meeting of these pioneers, and sixty people attended. Among them were Dr. John Hillabrand, Lore Maier, and Sister Paula Vandegaer. Most of the original sixty pioneers were Catholic, but they did not think of their work as "denominational." They thought of it as "humanitarian." (Monsignor McHugh also held two meetings in Washington for political and legislative pro-life activists well before January 22, 1973, and had thirty-five states represented. He used the name "National Right to Life," but gave this name to Dr. J. C. Willke and others when they eventually formed that nonprofit corporation.)

Out of that first meeting in early 1971, a follow-up one in Toronto (where it was proposed that all centers take the name of Birthright and adopt the same charter), and a mailed-in survey of participants, a new vision was birthed. It was a federation of independent alternatives to abortion service providers, quite different from each other, based in the United States, also networking with those outside our country who were catching the vision. This led quickly to our founding and the constitutional meeting of AAI held that same year, in November, in Chicago.

But the story of our founding and foundations is more than one of dates and events during the birth of the entire pro-life movement; it is a story of real and fascinating people with vision, values, and beliefs that are still an essential part of who Heartbeat is today.

Our Medical Roots:
John Hillabrand, M.D. (1908–1992)

Dr. John Hillabrand was born over a century ago. "Dr. John," as most others and I knew him, had been in medical practice for thirty-seven years before the founding of AAI in 1971. He received his medical degree from University of Michigan in 1934. He did residencies on obstetrics and gynecology at St. Vincent's Hospital in Toledo, Ohio, at Boston Lying-in Hospital, Boston, Massachusetts, and at the Illinois Research Hospital in Chicago, Illinois. He started private practice in Toledo in 1938, served four years in the U.S. Navy Medical Corps during World War II, and returned to Toledo in 1946, where he served the community until his reluctant retirement at age eighty-two.

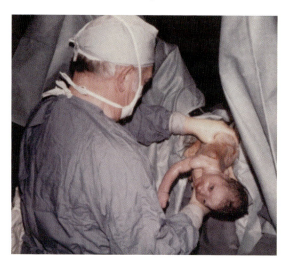

▲ *Dr. John ensures that one of his precious mothers has a healthy delivery. He often said that he had delivered more than eight thousand babies and never lost a mother.*

Dr. John was an obstetrician and gynecologist in solo-practice who had a personal care for each of his patients and who loved delivering babies. As a doctor and Catholic, his respect for human life was a natural part of him. For him, healing was both a physical and a spiritual calling. A snapshot of a beaming Dr. John and his wife from our files, with thirteen of their grandchildren (at that time all apparently under the age of about eight!), shows how much he valued family and children.

I heard him say more than once, "I have delivered more than eight thousand babies and never lost a mother." When I first heard him make that statement, after I had already become a part of the pro-life movement, I was sure he was going to finish the sentence with "never lost a baby." But his respect for life, and desire to protect and guard it, extended not only to babies but also, of course, to their mothers. And, in fact, to the mothers and babies equally and at the same time because he considered both to be his patients.

This was an essential perspective that Dr. John brought to AAI and that is still part of Heartbeat International today. We are both mother- and baby-centered. We do much more than "save babies." We save lives in a life-changing way, both for mothers and babies, and for others in the family circle as well. As our story proceeds, and AAI matures into Heartbeat International, this will be even more evident.

Dr. John spoke up publicly and became active when he saw his patients, either mothers or babies, in jeopardy. He saw the effects of the early doses of the birth control pill, whose high estrogen levels led to many deaths from blood clots. He became an expert witness in court cases relating to the pill in the 1960s, and was also an expert witness in appellate court cases of women who were severely injured by or died from "safe, legal" abortions after 1973. He was a consulting expert at annual meetings of the American Trial Lawyers Association in Dallas and in New York City.

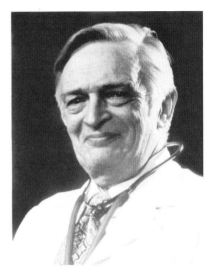

▲ Dr. John Hillabrand, M.D., founder of AAI. This is how most of those in AAI from the 1970s and 1980s would remember Dr. John.

He also understood, from a scientific and moral perspective, that human life begins at conception. So, when the drive to legalize abortion began, he testified in state legislatures and in Washington, D.C., on when human life begins and on what abortion actually consists of: the destruction of human life.

Recently, at a small event in a private home for Heartbeat International, one of the guests was Bob Marshall, a state representative in Virginia. When he realized that Heartbeat was the same organization that was started by Dr. John, he was eager to tell me his story. Over forty years ago, as a recent college graduate, he was hired as a legislative aide in Congress, and he was witness to the first hearings in our nation's capital on the question "When does human life begin?" He remembered Dr. John Hillabrand's persuasive testimony that human life begins at conception and must be respected and protected, and he told me how powerful Dr. John's debating skills were, as he demolished the vacuous arguments of pro-abortion proponents in Congress. Representative Marshall offered to send me copies of Dr. John's congressional testimonies that he kept in his office files all these years!

What a blessing it was for me to meet someone, so unexpectedly, who was as touched personally by Dr. John as I have been. If only our country had made truth, for which Dr. John was such a good witness, the basis for our laws and court decisions at that time, how much death and suffering would have been prevented.

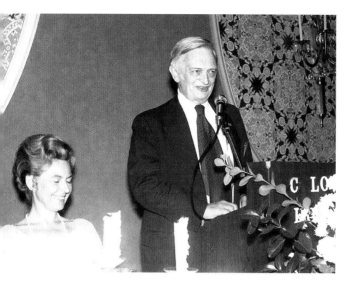

An outstanding practitioner in his field, Dr. Hillabrand was board-certified, a member of the American College of Surgeons and International College of Surgeons, and a member of fourteen other medical academies and societies. He was a founding fellow of the American College of Obstetricians and Gynecologists, but his convictions caused him to resign in 1973, in protest of their pro-abortion position.

▲ *Dr. John as M.C. at an early AAI Academy, introducing speaker Phyllis Schlafly, founder of Eagle Forum, which helped defeat the Equal Rights Amendment to the Constitution (that could have enshrined feminist-favored "rights" such as abortion).*

Dr. John naturally brought professionalism, emphasis on collegiality, and high standards into the foundation of AAI. This emphasis was prevalent in all the early meetings and conferences (called academies) of AAI and in all of his AAI communications, and it has become a core value of Heartbeat International.

Our terminology has changed: we called our movement then the E.P.S. movement, standing for Emergency Pregnancy Services. Today we call it the pregnancy help movement. We were then and still are today an association of independent affiliates (providing a wide range of services that are alternatives to abortion) who respect each other, learn from each other, and desire to do our work in a spirit of collegiality and entrepreneurialism, both challenging and collaborating with each other. We were then and are now grassroots and bottom up, not top down.

For example, this is what Dr. John wrote, in his elegant and somewhat formal style, in an invitation to the third annual AAI Academy in 1974. It is addressed to *"My Dear Friends in Service"*:

> *To state that the E.P.S. movement is glorious, humanitarian and unprecedented, has become a veritable cliché. Yet it is nonetheless true. It remains exciting, venturesome and rewarding. It is a grassroots movement by its very nature. It will never be a "trickle down" establishment where all the brains, inspiration, know-how and initiative are at the top. Every registrant is in fact a rich repository whose duty is to share earned experience with others who stand to profit therefrom.*

Dr. Hillabrand was a humble man, and he was always learning, as well as giving of his time and experience. With such a busy professional life, it is hard to imagine how he had the energy to start three of the very first national and international pro-life organizations that are still among the strongest and most influential pro-life groups. As well as being a co-founder of AAI, now Heartbeat International, he was also a founding member of Americans United for Life (also started in 1971), and he served as chairman of its executive committee. He also was program co-chairman of the first international pro-life meeting held in New York City in 1967, and was active in four subsequent international meetings until the National Right to Life Committee was formed and grassroots support was developed. (He also helped found Ohio Right to Life in 1968.)

In his own medical practice, Dr. John saw many women with unexpected, even "crisis," pregnancies. When abortion became legal in a few states, even before January 22, 1973, it was an option that women began to ask about, many feeling pressured to seek out abortion as the new "safe, legal" alternative.

Dr. John's longtime nurse and office manager, Esther Applegate, told me that many of his patients brought in nieces and friends who needed help and support. He would see them in his practice and then refer them to existing community services, but there were more girls and women in need than he and his office nurse could personally handle, especially with the care and attention he wanted them to have. Esther said, "He knew abortion was around the corner" and a bigger safety net was needed.

So, he decided to open another office, close to his medical practice and to call it "Heartbeat of Toledo." It was one of only a handful of pregnancy help centers in the country, and it opened its doors in 1971. Esther Applegate, who moved between the medical office of Dr. Hillabrand and the new pregnancy center, soon located in the same building, was helping girls and women in both locations. She remembers Dr. John's excitement and sense of humor on the opening day of this pioneering pregnancy center. Esther told me, with a smile, "He called on the phone the first day and tested us by saying, 'My daughter is pregnant and considering abortion, where can I take her?' But I recognized his voice!"

In the same year that Heartbeat of Toledo, Ohio, opened its doors, Dr. John attended that legendary meeting of sixty pioneers in Washington, D.C., and then the constitutional meeting of AAI in Chicago (where he was elected treasurer of the new organization).

Another person from Toledo, Mrs. Lore Maier, was also an important part of each of these three events of 1971.

Our Humanitarian Roots:
Lore Maier (1923–2004)

Mrs. Eleanore Maier, whom most people called Lore (pronounced Laura), was born in Germany in 1923 and barely lived through the Hitler era. She immigrated to the United States in 1951 and became a citizen in 1957. She has a fascinating and courageous story that helps explain her passion for the sanctity of human life and why she devoted so much of her life to serving mothers and babies and to the development of AAI, now Heartbeat International.

Lore was a ten-year-old student at the Lyceum of St. Therese in her native Loebschuetz, Germany (in Upper Silesia, now part of Poland), in 1934, when Hitler came to power. In an interview published in *The Catholic Chronicle*, May 20, 1983, Lore recounted many of the details of those years. At her school, crucifixes and religious pictures were removed. "You could see their eerie outlines on the walls," she recalled. Pictures of Hitler youth leaders were hung. The curriculum was changed, and lay teachers replaced the nuns one by one, until only two were left to mop the floors. Although Lore's father, a World War I cavalry officer, opposed the Nazis, she was forced to join the Hitler youth groups. "If you were a child who wasn't a Hitler supporter . . . you were often excluded from games and relationships with your peers." And police observers were everywhere.

She eventually followed her dream to study acting at the university, and she joined a community theater group in Danzig (where she took roles of heroic women, including Joan of Arc). But in 1944, the Russians began a final assault and she was in the path of the violence and chaos that accompanied the collapse of Nazi Germany. She had left Danzig at age twenty-one and returned to Loebschuetz to be with her mother and to try to save what was left of her family. Her father had died; her brother (conscripted into the German navy) had frozen to death in the waters off Finland after his submarine was torpedoed. Within a couple months of Lore's return to her hometown, her mother died. In February of 1945, she was able to get her pregnant sister out of Germany to have her baby, in relative safety, in Prague. Thus, Lore's own sister and her nephew were the first of many mothers and babies that Lore saved. Even so, she often referred to herself as her family's sole survivor of Nazi Germany.

▶ *Lore Maier, founder and first executive director of AAI.*

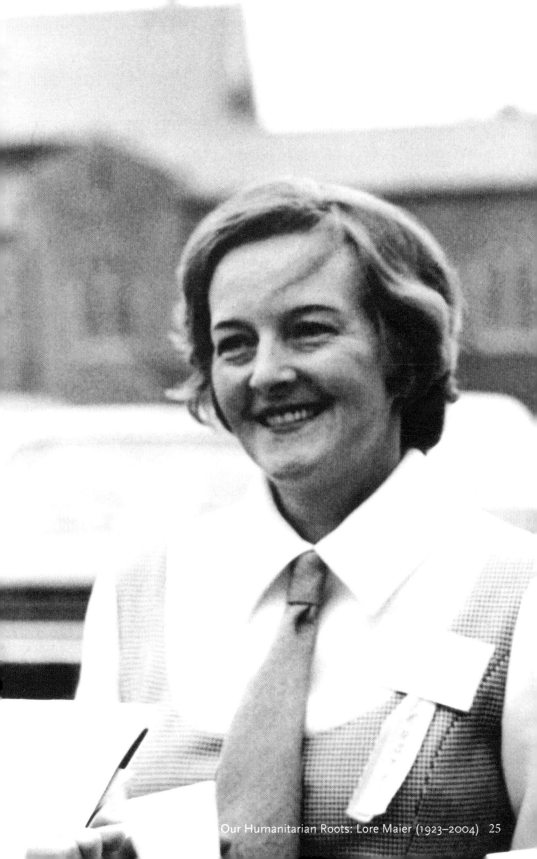

Lore recalled that when it was imminent that the Russians would come, refugees were fleeing the war and arriving in her city from Hungary, Romania, Russia, and elsewhere. "Women in open trucks clutched babies that had frozen to death." Prisoners freed from concentration camps arrived in the city. "There were long columns of gray-faced skeletons," she recalled. (Loebschuetz is not far from one of the most notorious death camps, Auschwitz, in Poland, and it is close to what was then the border of Czechoslovakia.) Lore brought some of the refugees into her family home and she refused to leave.

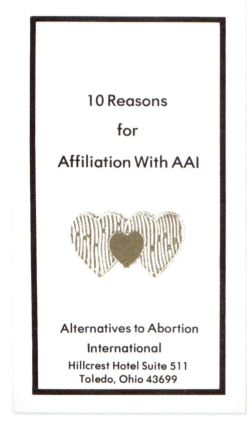

10 Reasons
for
Affiliation With AAI

Alternatives to Abortion
International
Hillcrest Hotel Suite 511
Toledo, Ohio 43699

▲ *One of the first AAI pamphlets, written by Lore Maier, featuring our original logo, the "Hearts of Gold," still incorporated in the current Heartbeat International logo.*

Loebscheutz changed hands between the Germans and the Russians five times. Finally, bombs were falling day and night and her house collapsed around her. She made it outside to find "human bodies and horse carcasses everywhere." She ran to the local hospital and volunteered with the Red Cross, helping wounded war victims and refugees of many nationalities. She eventually helped evacuate the city as the Russian army took over.

Then began a three-month harrowing journey. Lore, sometimes walking with bleeding feet, sometimes hiding and traveling in trucks or other vehicles, wandered with hoards of other refugees, with almost no food, out of Germany and through Czech territory (where the Czechs were welcoming the Russians). German nationals were being shot (sometimes by Czechs, sometimes by Russians). With the help of one German who spoke Czech, at one point she saved her life by posing as a Red Cross nurse on Czech business, using the only Czech word she knew, "Welcome."

She was interred in three different refugee camps, operated by Czechs, where the refugees had almost nothing to eat but thistles in the fields. "We were like goats; we picked the ground clean," she said. Conditions were so terrible that many died around her. Despite the threat that those who fled would be shot, she planned her escape. One rainy night, she hid in the women's latrine until 11 p.m., and then slid on her stomach under the barbed wire of the camp. She eventually made her way into Bavaria where, she said, "It was like coming out of hell. There were fields and people. Two American soldiers gave me my first American passport."

Lore stayed in postwar Bavaria and threw herself into humanitarian work. She worked with the United Nations Relief and Rehabilitation Administration, aiding concentration camp victims. Then for two years she worked for the Spruchkammer (Court of Justice), where she was a court reporter for the German government trials of Nazi war criminals. From 1949 to 1951, she was executive secretary of the Government Water Division in Munich, Germany.

Lore immigrated to the United States in 1951 and married Frederick Karl Maier, a United States citizen, in 1952. I understand that they met in the United States but returned to Germany for their marriage, then settled in Toledo, Ohio, where Mr. Maier owned a steel company. Lore became a citizen in 1957.

Lore said, in the interview from 1983, that her wartime experience left her with little bitterness. Rather, she said, it left her with a passionate interest in life and its protection. Her inspirational speeches and articles, published in some of the first pro-life publications, focus on the danger of violent solutions to perceived social problems, the intrinsic value of every human life, and the fact that, at least in the United States, we have the power to choose life, not death.

Although I met Lore at an Ohio Right to Life Convention in Columbus, Ohio, in 1978, an event that radically changed my direction in the pro-life movement (see introduction), I never knew the details of her past until I read them many years later from clippings in the AAI files. In my eyes, she was always a beautiful, elegant lady from the generation of my parents, the World War II or "Greatest Generation," who was a highly motivational and eloquent writer and speaker. I can vouch that not only did she have no bitterness, she was a very hopeful and inspirational leader who focused not on the past but only on a positive vision of the present and future. She often pointed out that people have the freedom (unlike in Nazi Germany) to make changes in the law, to recognize the sanctity of life of each person, and to engage in humanitarian service that could overcome the tide of abortion and disrespect for human life.

Later, I would come to realize that more was needed than humanitarian service and changes in the law. By the time I became Heartbeat International president in 1993, it was clear that the damage caused over twenty years (since 1973) by abortion on demand in our country, and caused worldwide by the lack of respect for human life, needed not only political and humanitarian action but also a cultural and spiritual "cure." This led to changes implemented as AAI became Heartbeat International in the 1990s. But that is the subject of a subsequent chapter in our history.

From our own experience since 1973, we recognize the effects of the lack of respect for human life not only on the victims but also on our society as a whole. Even before the *Roe v. Wade* decision, however, Lore warned us of what would happen to our culture (because she saw what had happened in Nazi Germany). Here are some of her words from an article in *Marriage and Family Newsletter*, April 1971, a publication with international subscriptions, edited by John E. Harrington. Lore's article, published along with letters from readers in London, Rome, Brazil, Canada, and the Philippines, was headlined, "If we are not pro-life we are against our own survival."

> *I lived comparatively close to Auschwitz, the concentration camp most infamous for the extermination of innocent prisoners. My townspeople never knew what was going on in there during the war. Whispers had been heard toward the end of the war, but the whole bitter truth did not come out until the prisoners were liberated and streamed in long columns through the streets of my little home town in their ragged uniforms. Their faces were numb and their spirit was gone in spite of their new freedom. Even in those victims who survived, the dehumanizing impact of destruction and cruelty was apparent. From the foregoing it is clear that inhuman behavior takes its toll not only from the victim, but also from the oppressor, as well as from those who stand by idly or helplessly in silent acquiescence.*

> *And so it is with abortion. The victim loses every time. The abortionist becomes emotionally detached and insensitive to the value of human life. The bystander, even though initially interested and concerned, may tire of the controversy and succumb to the semantic gymnastics and clever subterfuge of the proponents. Unknowingly, indifference gradually takes over to the point of complete apathy. The mother, because of her particular role, may suffer in one or all of these areas. Yet it is the mother who determines the fate of man. She holds society together or causes it to crumble, because she is the pillar, the mother of all men. . . .*

> *If we choose abortion, we will pay the highest price. Abortion is worse than war, worse than any inhumanities of any dictatorship, because it erodes the moral fabric of society . . . Abortion not only takes a far greater toll of innocent life, but it degrades the abortion collaborators to the lowest level of cruelty and immorality . . . Our efforts to push back the tide of abortion will be the measure of our character and will determine for us and for all posterity the kind of world in which we shall live.*

> *If we are not pro-life, we are against our own survival!*

How did this refugee from Nazi Germany go from being the immigrant wife of a successful Toledo businessman to a pioneer in the pro-life movement and a key ally of Dr. Hillabrand? Dr. John knew Mr. and Mrs. Maier, and Lore, who was one of his patients, he called Frau Maier. Dr. Hillabrand's nurse, Esther Applegate, recalls that Lore was widowed in 1967, after only fifteen years of marriage. She was childless. She was distraught and grieving, and entered into a period of depression. Dr. Hillabrand, needing help with his many pro-life endeavors and knowing Frau Maier's history and her organizational skills, said to Lore, "Do I have a job for you!"

So, Lore was "called" through another person who perceived her gifting and sensed that God might have a role for her. That is the story of most of us involved in this Great Work! The rest, as they say, is history. Lore was the co-founder with Dr. John of that early pregnancy center, Heartbeat of Toledo, and at one time was its executive director. She was one of the sixty people present in Washington, D.C., when the idea of a networking body or federation for the emerging centers was birthed. And she became the first executive director of AAI, chosen for this role at the constitutional meeting in Chicago in 1971.

In the 1970s, a formative decade for the entire pro-life movement, Lore was also a board member (for more than ten years) of AUL, Americans United for Life, in Chicago. She was also a co-founder and vice president of PLAN (Protect Life in All Nations), a world federation of international, national, regional, and professional pro-life organizations and foundations (started in Washington, D.C., in 1978). She also joined the Advisory Board of American Life Lobby, in Washington, D.C. Her strong belief in collaboration and unity, reflected in the founding vision of AAI and in her role with these other organizations, is still a core value of Heartbeat International.

Like Dr. John, Lore seemed to be a ball of energy, and she worked countless hours, all on a volunteer basis, to lay the foundations for several pro-life organizations, especially for AAI. As I look at the records from her tenure as executive director of AAI, whose first office was set up in Toledo, Ohio, I am amazed at the amount of work she produced with only a small cadre of equally passionate volunteers.

This was the era when electric typewriters were in vogue and Xerox technology was not widespread. Multiple copies of things were generally made from dittoes (with smeary, purple ink) or mimeograph. Thousands of pieces of paper are in the files from this period, including many carbon copies, lists that were painstakingly typed, retyped, and corrected (presumably drafted from index cards that were then alphabetized to help organize the hundreds of contacts that were being made around the world). There are hundreds, perhaps thousands, of personal letters that Lore composed and answered from throughout the United States and around the world.

The first list of centers in existence (called the *Directory*, now called the *Heartbeat International Worldwide Directory Desk Reference*) was developed by Lore and given to board members in 1972. It was distributed on mimeographed sheets of paper. It contained about 130 entries, including all the pregnancy centers known to exist in the United States (including those in the start-up phase), plus eleven in Canada and one in New Zealand.

Our present *Worldwide Directory* contains over 5,461 entries in eighty-seven countries. It is developed using the latest in database technology, and is available (and updated regularly) on the worldwide web. When I think of the work that Lore and her volunteers did to keep track of this fast-growing movement, with the now-primitive tools available, it is truly amazing!

Lore soon needed help in the office of AAI in Toledo, and she invited our third co-founder, Sister Paula Vandegaer, to move to Ohio from California to help her. Sister Paula declined, but she offered to open a west coast office for AAI in Los Angeles, and that was soon done.

Chapter 4

Our Roots in the Dignity of Women: Sister Paula Vandegaer, S.S.S.

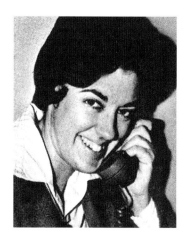

▲ *Sister Paula Vandegaer, founder of AAI, pictured in the late 1970s. Sister taught counseling skills, including counseling over a hotline.*

Our third co-founder, Sister Paula Vandegaer, S.S.S., a member of the Academy of Clinical Social Workers and a Licensed Clinical Social Worker in the state of California, is still active today, tirelessly answering the pro-life call that she responded to as a young member of a religious order, Sisters of Social Service. Today, forty years after she helped found AAI, Sister Paula is the active president of International Life Services, based in Los Angeles (which she also founded in 1985), which provides training and education on all aspects of the sanctity of human life, from conception to natural death.

She was recently honored at the Fortieth Anniversary Conference of Heartbeat International with the first of Heartbeat's "Legacy Awards." At its inauguration, this is the description of the award: "Heartbeat International's Legacy Awards recognize people within Heartbeat International who have made an outstanding contribution that not only has enriched our movement, but will be handed down to future generations." The legacy left to all of us and our movement from Sister Paula is her contribution to our founding principles and values, teaching resources, and professional standards.

Sister Paula created the first counseling manual in our field, even before AAI was founded. She applied the principles of professional counseling and social work to a brand new mission: crisis pregnancy "counseling" done by lay people providing alternatives to abortion. Sister Paula's original manual and her widespread trainings throughout the country resulted in the fact that, as Sister sometimes smilingly points out, there are parts of her early manual in almost every current pregnancy help training manual used today! However, in the late 1960s, when Sister took on this task, the field of crisis intervention for women was relatively new, and crisis phone lines were not common (early "crisis counseling" was done on groundbreaking suicide prevention hotlines). Moreover, a general standard of the profession of social work is "client self-determination," that is, the client must ultimately make her own choices. How does a Christian person in this new field of crisis counseling for pregnant women who could now choose abortion reconcile this professional standard with our conviction that the choice of abortion is not a good or ethical choice either for the woman or for her baby?

Sister Paula's pioneering manual and training articles (later published in the AAI magazine called *Heartbeat*) emphasized treating every woman who comes to us with a crisis pregnancy (or after abortion) with unconditional respect and love. She, a person created by God, must be the center of our attention and concern (not the occasion for a "lecture" from us or a debate on the pros and cons of abortion). Sister Paula always emphasized the importance of listening carefully to each woman's story and treating her in a loving, caring, and nonjudgmental way, the importance of discovering who she is, affirming her, and helping her discern the best choice for her baby and herself, based on who God created her to be as a woman (as Sister might say, the psychology of who she is as a woman and the difference between what abortion and motherhood will mean to her as a woman). Sister also emphasized that, while the woman will ultimately make the final decision on whether or not to have an abortion, she deserves complete information on abortion and its risks as well as complete information on the development of her baby.

How did Sister Paula Vandegaer come to leave such a legacy to our movement? Well, like anyone who has received a "call" on his or her life, because she said "yes" to the Lord, Sister's life took shape very differently from what she had originally planned. In fact, when I interviewed Sister Paula for our Fortieth Anniversary video and Legacy Award, she laughingly told me, "Three things I never wanted to be were a nun, a writer, or a teacher. And, I became all three!"

Sister took her vows as a member of the Sisters of Social Service as a young girl in 1959. She then earned a B.A. degree in psychology from Immaculate Heart College in Los Angeles, in 1962. She then went on for a Master's in Social Work from the Catholic University of America in Washington, D.C., specializing in Psychiatric Casework. She returned to Los Angeles and began working, from 1966 to 1968, as a caseworker for the Catholic Welfare Bureau, where she did general counseling of a wide variety of clients. The Lord began to specifically prepare her for what lay ahead when she became a supervisor and caseworker in the Natural Parent Department of Holy Family Services in Los Angeles, an adoption and pregnancy-counseling agency specializing in counseling unwed mothers and fathers.

At that time, agencies of the Catholic Church, especially Catholic Social Services agencies, were in the forefront of providing professional social work services related to crisis pregnancies. They operated many homes for unwed mothers and many adoption agencies across the country. Catholic Social Services agencies are still numerous and handle some related cases; however, the demand for maternity homes, especially large ones with related adoption agencies, has all but disappeared in the United States, due to the wide-spread promotion of abortion and the fact that unwed motherhood is no longer considered a stigma. In a sense, our volunteer-based pregnancy help movement, using lay "counselors" and other client advocates, and now nurses and other medical personnel, has largely replaced these

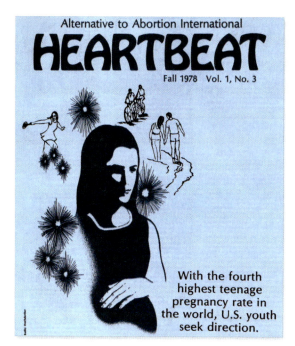

Alternative to Abortion International

HEARTBEAT

Fall 1978   Vol. 1, No. 3

With the fourth highest teenage pregnancy rate in the world, U.S. youth seek direction.

▲ *This is a sample of* Heartbeat *magazine, the first professional journal for our field, edited and published by Sister Paula from the West Coast Office of AAI from 1977 to 1986.*

formal social services for those facing a crisis pregnancy. And, Sister Paula gave lay people the tools, early in our movement, to help women in a professional, loving, and caring way.

Pro-abortion proponents began efforts to change the abortion law in California (and other states) in the mid-1960s. A loose coalition of pro-life people of various professions got together to fight this legislation and to lobby against the bill in the California legislature. They eventually called themselves the Right to Life League (believed to be the first pro-life group to organize in the United States and use the name "right to life," and one of the first to offer pregnancy help services). The group was in contact with another member of the Sisters of Social Service, Sister Rosemary Markum, who urged Sister Paula to get involved.

The California law passed, despite their efforts, and was signed by Governor Ronald Reagan, who later said it was the one decision he regretted about his record as California's governor. He said he was misled by the "hard cases" arguments related to rape, incest, and life of the mother. But once abortion became legal in California, it was clear that a safety net was needed for women, and pro-life people had to be trained to talk to women and help them choose alternatives to abortion.

For example, the very first pro-life pregnancy hotline came into existence on May 5, 1971, in Whittier, California, through the efforts of Margaret Nemecek, as an outreach of the Right to Life League of Southern California. Sister Paula, then a board member of the Right to Life League, was asked to train the first hotline workers who were members of Margaret's daughter's Girl Scout troup!

Sister Paula gathered together four social workers from Catholic Social Services (that has always had a policy that their counselors do not refer for abortions), and they met every two weeks for three months to develop that first training manual. Right to Life League began doing pregnancy tests at the Whittier center soon after that, and the League became one of the first affiliates of AAI when we were formed in 1971, with leadership from Sister Paula.

On a personal note, it is amazing for me to realize that I (an "Ohio girl") was in college for four years, in California, at this same time (see introduction). I saw the billboards advertising abortion services going up, and I was shocked and appalled. I had no idea until many years later that the pro-life movement was also developing in that state at that very same time, and that someday I would be carrying on the work of one of the California founders of this movement, Sister Paula Vandegaer.

Sister Paula first met Dr. John and Lore at that 1971 meeting in Washington, D.C., and the follow-up meeting in Toronto. She recalls that the three of them and others sat up until 2:00 a.m. debating whether a franchise model (as was proposed) would work in the United States, where a variety of diverse service models for pregnancy centers were already being used. Sister says that after that meeting, Lore Maier and Dr. John, who had been appointed to help organize efforts in the United States, sent out a questionnaire to all the U.S. groups in attendance. The overwhelming desire was for a federation model of independent service providers, not a franchise model.

According to Sister, Lore and Dr. John worked very quickly after that to develop this new organization, their work culminating in the constitutional meeting in November of 1971 in Chicago, and the naming of this new group AAI. Sister Paula could not make it to Chicago for this first meeting, but came to the second board meeting in early 1972 and was promptly elected secretary of AAI. At that meeting, Lore distributed that first list of centers and contact persons interested in starting a center in the United States with about 130 names.

At that point, Sister Paula became the right-hand person to Lore Maier. Lore promptly wrote a manual called *Suggested Guidelines for Establishing Pro-Life Emergency Pregnancy Service (E.P.S.) Centers*. Along with Sister's *Pregnancy Counseling Manual*, people with a passion for the mission had everything they needed to get going! Sister recalled, "It was so exciting to see all the energy—the Holy Spirit was moving throughout the land, and all before 1973! Once we had the manuals, from then on it went like crazy—centers were starting at a rate of two per week! The movement was so rapid, so incredible. I was traveling all over to give trainings, from New York to Hawaii. Our feeling was, for God's sake, get them going."

Like most of us who have come later into this same movement, Sister Paula found out that God does not call the equipped, he equips the called. To show His power and build our faith, He asked her to step out of her comfort zone of professional counseling and depend on Him. She told me an amazing story of how, at a crucial point in our history, the Lord provided her a vision, made it perfectly clear that the vision was from Him, and then brought her the help and tools she needed to make that vision a reality.

Lore needed more help in the office in Toledo and asked Sister to move there and assist her. However, Sister had a role in her religious order and could not leave California. She saw that she could help Lore by taking over the newsletter. It consisted of mimeographed sheets that were sent out monthly to all centers and other contacts. But she also knew that the newsletter needed a major upgrade; in fact, she realized that it could and should be an informative and professional journal or magazine for our field. (Right to Life had just begun their newsletter, the first and only one for pro-life at that time.) Sister was trained how to counsel, but she knew nothing about writing and publishing a magazine. Yet, she thought that this was exactly what God wanted her to do!

God gave her several unmistakable signs as a confirmation. First, one of the younger Sisters said that her brother, former editor of his college newspaper, wanted a job in publishing and he was willing (for a small salary) to edit and publish the magazine for them. Sister knew she would have to raise some money. After a meeting, she was putting some dishes away and chatting with those present. She began to share the vision. One woman gave her $5,000, and a priest gave her $1,000. She did a phone-a-thon soon after and quickly raised all the funds she would need for the first year!

The brother designed a brochure for Sister Paula to use in selling the idea to the AAI Board, but he left a hole in the brochure for a picture, to be added later. He went on vacation, leaving Sister to fill that hole. Sister remembers walking down a hallway, thinking and praying to herself, "God,

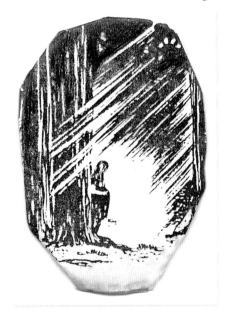

▲ Image of the pregnant girl in a dark wood, with rays of light representing the hope that the church can bring to those in distress. This is Kathy's original drawing for the brochure promoting Heartbeat magazine. It was inspired by her dream and her friend Karen, who committed suicide after an abortion.

I don't know how to write, I know nothing about printing, I know nothing about all of this—I am a social worker!"

Sister soon ran into an old friend named Kathy Hochderfser, an artist, who knew nothing, from Sister, about the idea of the magazine or how inadequate Sister was feeling. Kathy mentioned to Sister Paula that she recently had a dream about her. In her dream, Kathy and another artist friend were in a room with Sister Paula, who was pacing back and forth. Kathy told Sister Paula, in the dream, "Sit down and stop worrying. We are laying out the magazine for you."

When Sister recovered somewhat from her shock in hearing the dream, she asked Kathy if she knew who the other person was in the dream. Kathy said that the other person in the dream was Karen, who had painted with her many years ago. Karen had been raped as a girl, and her mother had forced her to have an abortion. She became so distraught over the abortion that, many years later, she shot herself in the head.

Dumbfounded, Sister was finally able to tell Kathy about her vision for the magazine to help the fledgling alternatives to abortion movement, and about the urgency of the brochure with the hole in it! Kathy immediately offered to help, but she confessed that she had no idea what to draw for that brochure. It would have to be a key image to convey the vision. Sister asked Kathy to pray about it overnight.

The next day Kathy returned with a sketch of a pregnant girl, leaning against a tree in a dark forest, but there were rays of light filtering through the darkness. There was the bare hint, at her feet, of sticks fallen in the form of a cross. It seemed inspired! This was the picture that was added to the "hole" in the brochure. Sister took this to the board meeting in Pittsburgh in 1977, and the board approved the idea of the magazine, as well as the founding of the West Coast office of AAI (Sister Paula's office), where the magazine would be published.

The Lord used Sister Paula and *Heartbeat* magazine to help bring about the phenomenal growth and development of the pregnancy help movement. And, given the central role of Karen in Kathy's dream and perhaps in the inspiration for the girl in the woods, it is fitting that *Heartbeat* magazine published the first research in the entire pro-life movement suggesting the existence of post-abortion syndrome (in a study from Japan). And it is also fitting that the movement Sister Paula helped found also birthed many of the first abortion recovery programs (and 82 percent of current Heartbeat affiliates have such programs as part of their core services).

But that is not the end of the story of how the Lord confirmed Sister's mission. At a subsequent AAI Academy, the keynote speaker was Archbishop Elko. He told them about an experience he had had many years before on a train in Europe. A young man came into his compartment and said, "You're a priest, aren't you. I hate the church." The man then spent the rest of his time in the compartment sketching on a pad. When he came to his stop, he tore the drawing off the pad and gave it to the Bishop. It was a picture of a young woman in a forest, leaning against a tree, but there was no light. Departing the train, the young man said, "That's why I hate the church—the church puts you in dark places and does not show you a way out!" Sister Paula said that the Bishop's message to the audience was this: you, in the pro-life pregnancy help movement, are the light in the forest and YOU show women the way out.

Sister shared with me how awed she was that God had put together a woman who died many years before and an archbishop to help her see that He was in charge and would provide not only the vision but the means to make it a reality! She is also grateful that the Lord sent Kathy to her. Kathy was called into the pro-life movement on the day that she shared her dream with Sister Paula in 1977. She has been with Sister Paula ever since, first as the editor of *Heartbeat* magazine and now, thirty-four years later, as the executive director of International Life Services.

I was fortunate that Sister told me this story while we were sitting in her International Life Services office in Los Angeles. She was sitting very close to the drawing of the girl in the forest, with the light shining through the trees, the suggestion of the cross at her feet. A small version is on her desk, and a larger one is the only decoration on the wall. She sees this "lesson" again every day: we in the pregnancy help movement are the church, the Body of Christ, and the church does bring light in the darkness.

I feel fortunate that I was among the thousands of others who were trained by Sister Paula, year after year at the AAI Academies, from 1979 through the eighties, and who used her training and articles in *Heartbeat* magazine to guide my "counseling" with pregnancy center clients. Two of her key writings at that time for me were "Helping a Sexually Active Woman to Say 'NO'" and "The Guidance of the Spirit in Our Counseling." I used to take these two articles into the room with me while I waited for the results of the client's pregnancy test (this was before centers began "self-testing" and before we had medical clinics), and I read these articles over and over to give me insight and courage before I went out again to talk to the client.

This was in the early 1980s. When a client had a negative pregnancy test (over 50 percent of our tests were negative), it was tempting to simply give her the results and let her go, because our main purpose was to provide a safety net if the client had a positive test and was considering abortion. What to say to a girl or woman who was not pregnant at that point? We did not refer her for contraceptives, and, amazingly, we did not talk much about sexually transmitted diseases because there were basically only two (that we knew of) and they could be cured by antibiotics. Imagine the days before we even knew about HIV/AIDS! (It was in 1981 that researchers in San Francisco made note of a new and deadly illness among the gay population in San Francisco.)

Feminism was at its height, and I expected most girls and women might laugh at me if I suggested simply abstinence until marriage, especially at our pregnancy center office at the campus of The Ohio State University (where students sometimes came in with bizarre make-up and other attempts to show their rebellion from traditional norms and standards).

But Sister's articles gave me the courage to present my client a new vision of herself and her gift of sexuality, and ask her to consider a new way of life that was in keeping with the woman God created her to be. I'm sure I am not the only pregnancy center volunteer who was so affected by Sister's writings. My growing commitment to this vision of true womanhood eventually led to the development of the Sexual Integrity™ Program for Heartbeat International, to be discussed at the proper time in our history.

Sister Paula's emphasis on the dignity of the woman (from her psychological perspective) corresponded to Dr. Hillabrand's emphasis on caring for the woman (from his medical perspective), and these corresponded with Lore Maier's passion for the dignity of every human person (from her humanistic and experiential perspective). Underlying all these perspectives was the Christian faith of each of our founders, an essential part of who they were and how they viewed the world and those in it. This was true of all the pioneers in the pro-life movement. It was so integral to who they were that, paradoxically, they did not talk or write about it as explicitly as you might expect. This changed later in our movement, something that we will discuss as our history continues into the 1980s and 1990s.

Standing the Test of Time

Each of our three co-founders, Dr. John Hillabrand, Lore Maier, and Sister Paula Vandegaer, brought special gifts to our movement and to the establishment of AAI. They incorporated into our work the values, purposes, and principles that characterized not only our first twenty years but also that have undergirded the growth and development of Heartbeat International and the changes we have undergone, especially in the last twenty years. This chapter highlights, one by one, those values and principles that are standing the test of time.

Even More than Saving Babies

All three of our co-founders had a view of our work that encompassed more than "saving babies." Those who describe the mission of pregnancy help centers as saving babies are only describing a part of our founders' vision and mission. They focused on both mother and baby and, in fact, on the family and the entire culture. They saw that we were involved in this work to serve women in need and help them so they could save their babies, but also (especially in the work of Sister Paula) we were in a position to help women understand their true womanhood. Dr. John's and Lore's writings and talks also show that they viewed an attack on the sanctity of human life in the womb as an attack on all humanity and on society as a whole that would have profound ramifications. Lore tried to warn of the effect not only on women themselves and the family, but also on the perpetrators, and even on those who stood by and observed.

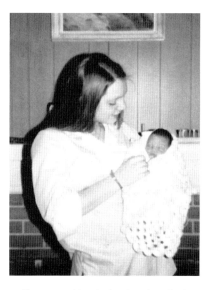

▲ Raena and her baby daughter in the 1970s. Dr. John Hillabrand delivered Raena's baby. Raena was a client of Lore Maier's and volunteered in the AAI office during her pregnancy. She made an adoption plan for her baby. Raena shared her story with Heartbeat just in time for our fortieth anniversary, an opportunity to honor our founders and the example they have left for our pregnancy help movement.

The first logo that was chosen for AAI, and that was used in the very first communications in early 1972, is still a part of the Heartbeat International logo. We recently chose it as the emblem of our Legacy Award. It is not a baby, nor is it a mother and child. It has always been called the

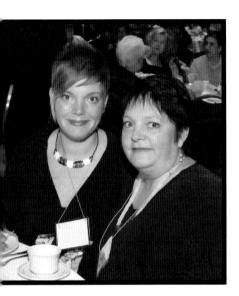

▲ At Heartbeat's fortieth anniversary banquet, Raena is with the daughter she placed for adoption in the 1970s, Shannon. They finally met again several years ago. Lore Maier's courage in Nazi Germany inspired Raena so much that she refused an abortion, against everyone's advice, when she became pregnant from rape, eight years after Shannon was born. Lore and Dr. John never knew about Raena's second pregnancy and her second daughter, Brienna.

"Hearts of Gold": two larger hearts with some lines and markings (the result of life's scars and experience, but also marks of maturity and wisdom) surround the tiny, unmarked, pure gold heart in the middle that represents the innocent human child. We need to protect, shelter, and nurture that child, born or unborn. The Hearts of Gold represent the family as God intended it. With the family disrupted and in need of healing, sometimes the larger, sheltering hearts are those of us in this movement, sheltering and protecting the child.

Collegiality

One of the primary values that our founders imbedded into Heartbeat was collegiality. It involves collaboration, respect for different ways of arriving at the same end, encouragement for the sharing of ideas, entrepreneurialism, constant improvement, and doing things in even more excellent and effective ways. This could also be expressed as unity within diversity.

This is reflected, first, in the structure of AAI as a federation of independent providers of alternative to abortion services. They are not all franchises of a particular model (although some may be). Our founders sometimes described AAI as a trade association for those called into the same work. This is true of Heartbeat International today, and thus we describe it as an "association" for those engaged in life-affirming service who voluntarily affiliate with each other under the banner of Heartbeat.

The value of collegiality, with an aim to constantly learn and improve, is also reflected in the annual training conference, begun by our founders as the annual AAI Academy and now called the Heartbeat International Annual Conference. Every year, for forty years, the affiliates of our organization have come together to teach and learn from each other. Presentations are given in large part by our own affiliates who can send a proposal for a workshop or presentation.

Heartbeat International is a "bottom up" organization not a "top down" one. While our central office now organizes the annual training events, for over twenty years of our history, the academies were hosted and planned almost entirely by individual affiliated organizations. Each year, one of the affiliates offered to host the conference in its home city, plan the program (with some help from the central office), design the conference brochure, and handle all the local arrangements for conference attendees. I have attended almost every conference since my first in 1979, and I can attest to the quality of those gatherings, planned and hosted by local centers (then) or with local centers (today) in a spirit of collegiality.

Principles of Affiliation

Other core values are expressed in our affiliation principles (that must be agreed to upon affiliation or re-affiliation). The original six were adopted early on by AAI. The first five of those are listed below. From the beginning, we have adopted the mentality expressed by Augustine of Hippo when he wrote, "In essential things unity, in forms and expressions freedom, over all things love."

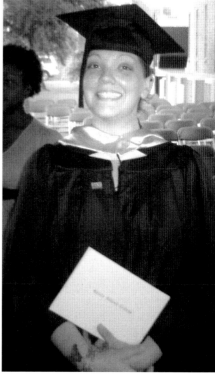

1. AAI affiliates propose and offer through education, action, and creative services, alternatives to abortion, and thereby provide positive choices for the woman distressed by pregnancy.
2. AAI affiliates shall not discriminate regarding race, creed, color, national origin, age, or marital status.
3. Services of AAI affiliates are personal and confidential.
4. AAI is nonjudgmental.
5. AAI affiliates shall not advise, provide or refer for abortion or abortifacients.

▲ *Brienna, Raena's second daughter, who was also saved through the love of our founders, Dr. John and Lore, and the courage of her mother, Raena.*

The original sixth principle was this: "AAI as an organization, takes no position with respect to political, religious, or family planning issues." When we became Heartbeat International in 1993, we decided to change this principle to indicate that Heartbeat affiliates "encourage chastity as a positive lifestyle choice." This was done because we thought the earlier principle could be misinterpreted or confusing. Abortion had become a political, religious, and family planning issue, and our programs certainly took a position against abortion. Meanwhile, we wanted to make it clear that we did take a position on chastity, defined as sexual purity both before marriage and within marriage (faithfulness to one's spouse).

Heartbeat's principles, adopted in 1993, are also the basis for the ethical principles first adopted in January 2001 by our entire pregnancy help movement, called Our Commitment of Care.

Heartbeat later led in the expansion of Our Commitment of Care to become Our Commitment of Care and Competence that was adopted by the entire pregnancy help movement in 2009. This commitment is included in appendix VI. The origin of this important statement of ethical principles is discussed in chapter 10.

Purpose of Central Office and Leadership

The original purposes of the central office of AAI, the services provided today to our member affiliates by the national/international office, were envisioned by our founders. Their list of what was needed was accurate, as evidenced by the fact that Heartbeat International still provides these core services (although other essential services have been added, as needs have grown, which will be noted further in our history). The list of services established by AAI founders is as follows:

1. Training resources
2. A regular newsletter
3. Consultation and training on site
4. An annual conference to share ideas and programs
5. A directory of all existing pregnancy help services
6. A toll-free number to help connect women in need with a pregnancy center

Our founders quickly were able to implement the first five of these six goals, but the last one, a grand vision of Lore Maier, was one that she never saw accomplished in her lifetime. Thirty-two years after our founding, however, in 2003, Heartbeat entered into a joint venture that birthed Option Line, the 24/7 call center that now handles approximately 240,000 contacts each year (phone calls, emails, instant messages, and chats) and refers these contacts to pregnancy help centers. I am happy to report that all our founders' entire vision (and more!) is being implemented, and the work is bearing fruit, through the Lord's grace and the army of love that the Lord has raised up.

International Affiliation

Another vision of our founders has become essential to who Heartbeat International is today. That is, their international vision. Almost immediately after the name AAI was adopted (Alternatives to Abortion Incorporated), Lore and Dr. John proposed that the initials AAI represent a new name, Alternatives to Abortion International. The board finally approved this change in 1974.

Lore, the executive director, in particular, had an international vision, coming as she did from Europe and speaking several languages. Her correspondence files show that she was exchanging letters, in the first few years of our history, with contacts from all over the world, urging them to start pregnancy help centers and keeping track of the nascent movement worldwide.

The official AAI directory of centers around the world, dated July 20, 1976, shows nine official affiliates, having been sent certificates of affiliation, outside the United States: three in Canada (Hamilton and Sudbury, Ontario, and Winnipeg, Manitoba); and one each in Auckland, New

Zealand; Amsterdam, The Netherlands; Bogota, Colombia; Everard Park, South Australia; Bern, Switzerland; and Port-Au-Prince, Haiti. Meanwhile, Lore had developed a World Council, an advisory board consisting of pro-life leaders in at least twenty other countries.

During Lore's tenure as executive director, she and Dr. John took many trips to other countries and continents, at their personal expense, to share the vision and consult with the growing network. Through the first twenty years of our history, the numbers of centers opening around the world continued to increase dramatically. AAI tried to keep track of the existence of all of them (whether or not they formally affiliated) through the regularly updated AAI directory.

International representatives often joined the AAI Board, the first one being Pierre Prineau from Bogota, Colombia; Daniel Overduin from Australia joined the board in 1977. When I joined the AAI Board in 1986, Bente Haugen from Norway was a fellow member. AAI Board minutes from 1977 indicate that AAI was aware of 782 centers in the United States and 1,350 foreign centers ("centers" at that point were often in the very beginning stage of formation).

Personal Involvement and Love

Our founders helped motivate and raise up thousands of people, mostly volunteers, around the world, whose primary tool or "weapon" for saving and changing lives was love, presented to clients in the form of personal involvement with them in their struggles. We now call that "cross bearing for the child-bearing." In a sense, our pioneers were fortunate in that they were not confused into thinking that there was a magic formula (some special protocol, picture, video, or even a tool like ultrasound—all invented much later and brought into the pregnancy center world from the 1980s on) that they could use to help the mother and save a baby's life.

We do have a lot of wonderful tools today, but they do not work very well unless incorporated with the personal touch, the personal involvement and love of one person shared with another. This takes time and sacrifice of self on the part of the person doing the loving. Human nature has not changed. God created us with a deep need to love and be loved, and most people respond with love and respect when they are treated in that manner. Even if they do not respond, our call to love remains.

That this was modeled by our founders and became a hallmark of AAI was evident when Heartbeat was contacted earlier this year by one of Dr. Hillabrand's and Lore Maier's original clients from the 1970s, Raena Avalon, who now lives in Sedona, Arizona. We had placed an invitation on our website for people to share their stories with us. Imagine our shock when the first person to communicate her story was Raena, who met Dr. John and Lore at Heartbeat of Toledo, Ohio, when she was sixteen and pregnant.

Raena told us that she has never forgotten the love and care that Dr. John and Lore had given her. She remembered that their original pregnancy help center was called Heartbeat. She was thinking of them one night, wishing she could "give back" some of what they gave her, so she googled

"Heartbeat" and found Heartbeat International! Here is Raena's original message to us about the love she received, a love that saved not just one baby, but two people:

In 1975 I found myself pregnant and alone. My father was a Baptist Minister and connected me with Dr. John Hillabrand in Toledo, Ohio. He and Lore Maier counseled me and convinced me to have the baby and Dr. Hillabrand became my obstetrician. I was close to eight months pregnant and had just had my first Lamaze class. One day I began to have terrible pains in my back. Dr. Hillabrand told me to meet him at his office. He announced, "We are having a baby!" I was five centimeters dilated, so he told us to get to the hospital. I was in the hospital about 1½ hours when he took me into the delivery room. He delivered my daughter slowly and gently. I wanted to keep her more than anything. I held her, and fed her and she smiled at me. I knew I couldn't provide for her or give her more than love and she needed much more than that. It was a chilly March day, my parents and I went to the church and on the altar we dedicated her to God and to his keeping. Then we took her to the Lutheran Social Services and I placed her for adoption.

After that I was so distraught and sad . . . I finished high school and went to a year of college. I then followed my parents to Rhode Island where my father had taken a new church. By the age of 23, I had become an alcoholic. I was homeless, sleeping in the city park with my clothes in a bus station locker. By the grace of God I got sober. At about two weeks of sobriety, I was raped. I was so hysterical and out of my mind that I went into a rehabilitation center. . . . They must have noticed something, because they made me take a pregnancy test. The results showed that I was pregnant and it could only be from the rape.

This time everyone insisted I had to have an abortion, that there was no way I could have the baby. Dr. Hillabrand and Lore Maier had a profound effect on me and made my dilemma of what to do with the growing fetus inside of me extremely difficult. I was praying and meditating on my bunk bed at the center and two men in white came into my mind. They told me that I was going to have another girl and that she was a gift from God. . . . They gave me her name and said that she had come just for me and that I would keep her and raise her as my own. She is 26 now and a beautiful ray of light in this world. She just got her MSW degree and majored in policy and homelessness.

The daughter I placed for adoption is 34 now and found me 14 years ago. She has wonderful adoptive parents and had a very good upbringing. She and I are very close and speak several times a month. She is so much like me and my other daughter that it is uncanny. I will always be grateful to Dr. John Hillabrand and to Lore Maier for their deep belief in the value of Life and for inspiring that quality in me.

When I called Raena on the phone and eventually met her in person in Sedona, she told me that her two daughters, neither born in ideal circumstances, "light up a room" when they enter! Both of them are involved in professions that "give back," and she cannot imagine the world without them. She confirmed that neither Dr. John nor Lore ever knew that the love they showed her when she was sixteen and pregnant with Shannon had also saved Brienna.

Raena told me that her father, the pastor, often dropped her off at Dr. John's office for a medical appointment, and then she would help Lore in the nearby AAI administrative office. Lore put her arm around her at one point, told her about her harrowing experiences in Nazi Germany, assured her that God had protected her, and that He would protect Raena as well. Raena told me that this was the message she remembered when she realized she was pregnant as a result of the rape: "If Lore had the courage and faith to go on, I can too. And God will help me."

Nondenominational

Finally, our three co-founders were Catholic. They were adamant, like all early pro-life leaders, that the movement not become solely a Catholic movement. In fact, our opponents did try to characterize it as such, to cause it to become marginalized and viewed as simply a reaction from a minority religious group that took its marching orders from celibate men in Rome. I personally heard these charges when I entered the movement in 1973. As our history shows, the Catholic hierarchy prodded the laity to get organized (as the meetings called by Monsignor McHugh demonstrate), but the official Catholic Church wanted only to be a catalyst for a broader movement of the Christian church, the Body of Christ.

The Catholic pro-life pioneers were very eager to get other Christians involved and into leadership. A recent article on the founding of the Evangelical pro-life organization originally called Christian Action Council or CAC, now Care Net, indicates that it was Catholic prompting and funding that launched their efforts as well. (The article was written by Robert Case, the first executive director of CAC, and published on ReformationArt.com.) At one point, CAC contacted AAI and asked for help and advice on starting pregnancy centers with an Evangelical statement of faith. The AAI Board invited the second executive director of that organization, Curtis Young, to serve on our board and learn everything he could from us. He did serve on the AAI Board in 1981 and 1982, and Christian Action Council "planted" their first Evangelical center in Baltimore in 1981.

Our founders adopted the terms "nondenominational and nonsectarian" to describe the nature of AAI. Lore Maier often used the term "humanitarian" to describe our work. (She had devoted herself to World War II–related missions, like the Red Cross and relief and resettlement services that were commonly described as "humanitarian.") To the affiliates, the meaning of these terms and how they applied to our services were never totally clear. Some affiliates interpreted them to mean (as I did, when my husband and I started our center in Columbus, Ohio, and affiliated with AAI) that we were not part of one denomination and would welcome all Christians to join us in this work.

Others interpreted the terms as meaning that it was inappropriate to "proselytize" or try to convert clients to our own beliefs. Still others seemed to think that these terms meant that AAI affiliates could not describe our organizations as "Christian" per se (nor as Catholic, Baptist, etc.), nor could we provide materials with a specific Christian message if we wanted to remain "nondenominational and nonsectarian." The lack of clarity on how to interpret these key terms led to great diversity among affiliates on how they viewed their identity: as a Christian organization or secular organization run by Christian people.

This part of our history and what it meant for our future was one of the major issues I needed to tackle when I became president in 1993. The culture had changed dramatically in the twenty-two years since our founding and was becoming more hostile to Christians. Our affiliates had changed, "denominational" centers like the Evangelical ones started by CAC now existed, and in many centers Catholics, Evangelicals, and other Christians were working closely together. The "second wave" of Evangelical Christians had joined our movement and was merging into the Catholic "first wave." The confusion over our "nondenominational and nonsectarian" identity, and how that was resolved, will be covered in the next section of our history.

Transition from the Founders

By 1985, our founders were no longer actively involved in the management and programming of AAI, and the central organization entered a period of decline. This is a somewhat predictable stage of development for organizations, once the initial period of rapid growth and development, fueled by the passion of the founders, comes to an end. The momentum could not be sustained, and a succession plan was not intentionally developed and implemented.

No doubt, spiritual attack had something to do with it too. The army was growing by leaps and bounds, and millions of people were hearing the message of love around the world. At the same

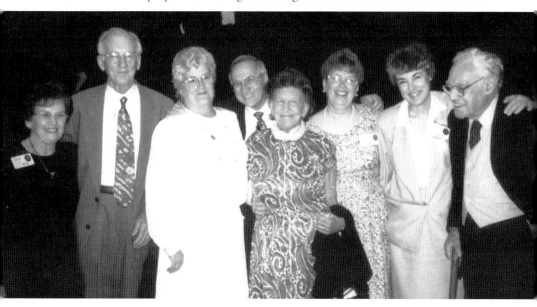

▲ Some of the founders of AAI and early leaders of our movement gathered in 1996 at the Twenty-Fifth Anniversary celebration of Heartbeat International in Chicago. Heartbeat's Servant Leader Award was inaugurated at this time, and the first awards were given to these individuals. Each year since, several foot soldiers within our movement, especially directors of our pregnancy help ministries, are honored with the Servant Leader Award. Pictured, L to R: Alice Brown (early chairperson of AAI Board), Frank Brown, Annette Krycinski (longtime secretary of the board), Thomas Krycinski, Margaret White, M.D., M.P. (one of the founders of SPUC, the first pro-life organization in the world, in England), Anne Pierson (Loving and Caring), Sr. Paula Vandegaer, Herb Ratner (best friend of Dr. John Hillabrand and present at the AAI constitutional meeting in 1971).

time, Planned Parenthood and its allies were increasing their stronghold on American culture and on international policy through the United Nations. Ronald Reagan's pro-life administration in the 1980s was, in retrospect, holding back the pro-abortion tide that broke through again during the Clinton administration.

Board minutes indicate some splintering among leadership, and they record misunderstandings that led to confusion and lack of unity. Another difficult issue was funding, which was always precarious for the central office. Affiliation fees had been reluctantly added but were a nominal $25 per center; the AAI directory was free, and an annual subscription to *Heartbeat* magazine was only $15 per year. Dr. John and Lore had been underwriting much of the budget for the central office in Toledo, and Sister Paula had borrowed from family and friends to make ends meet at the West Coast office.

Lore Maier announced her resignation as executive director in 1982, and Elinor Martin, founder of an excellent maternity home and center in White Plains, New York (now called the Elinor Martin Home), was appointed as executive director of AAI in 1983. She moved the administrative office from Toledo, Ohio, to White Plains. Sister Paula, who had operated the West Coast office of AAI and published *Heartbeat* magazine there, resigned in 1985. The West Coast office was closed and Sister founded International Life Services that she still heads today. Dr. John and Lore were both aging, but they continued to care deeply about the organization and the movement, and they stayed on the board through 1990.

Between 1985 and 1990, there were many changes in leadership, both on the staff and board, but the normal services that affiliates expected did continue: an annual Academy, an annual AAI directory, and *Heartbeat* magazine, now edited and published by an affiliate in Michigan. Unfortunately, Elinor Martin died, seemingly suddenly, from breast cancer. Her administrative assistant, Ellen Walsh, assumed the duties of executive director. The affiliate that I headed up in Columbus, Ohio, as chairman of the board, would have been somewhat unaware of the changes in leadership except that we had offered to plan and host the 1986 Academy with the theme "One Body, Many Members." Our written guidelines from AAI indicated that we needed input from the executive director, Elinor Martin, but because of her illness, she was unable to communicate with us, and we planned the program entirely on our own. After the conference, in fall of 1986, I was asked to join the AAI Board, and it was at that time that I understood the transition that we were experiencing.

In late 1988, Judy Peterson, who founded an outstanding maternity home in Orlando, called Beta, assumed the position of chairman of the board, Ellen Walsh resigned, and Judy's right-hand person in Orlando, Martha Scarito, became the executive director. Judy's vision involved major changes for AAI that included eliminating the AAI directory, de-emphasizing our international mission, changing our name to WHEF (Women's Health and Education Foundation), and making *Heartbeat* magazine a publication for young mothers, supported by advertising. The board members did not accept the new vision. We remained committed to the vision of our founders, and Judy resigned as chairman of the board in late 1989.

When Judy's resignation became known, board members were in phone contact with each other. I rented a meeting room at the Toledo Airport for a special board meeting in early 1990, within driving distance for some board members, and others agreed to fly in. Several board members resigned, due to age, family health problems, or general discouragement, leaving five of us: Lore Maier, Dr. John Hillabrand, Bente Haugen from Norway (not present), Carol McMahon from our affiliate maternity home Genesis, in Pittsburgh, and myself, from Pregnancy Distress Center, in Columbus. Carol was in the throes of planning our annual conference, hosted by her organization that year, so she could not assume additional duties (her husband died of a heart attack soon after and Carol had to resign from the board), and Dr. John and Lore had insisted on more of an advisory role.

I could not believe that the Lord would want AAI to simply cease to exist, having worked so powerfully through this organization for so many years. I saw that I was the sole person there who was in any position to take leadership. My respect for Dr. John and Lore and my passion for our mission would not allow me to do nothing. I offered to assume the role of "acting chairman of the board" and try to build up our board membership and find our next executive director. Still chairman of the board of our AAI affiliate in Columbus, I offered to move the administrative office to Columbus and be sure that we issued our AAI directory that year as well as a series of newsletters to keep our affiliates updated (to substitute for *Heartbeat* magazine), and that we recruited a host center for the next conference after Pittsburgh. Thus we could fulfill our basic commitment to affiliates as we rebuilt our infrastructure.

I came home to Columbus and called our previous offices in Orlando and White Plains to have our assets sent to Columbus. Orlando informed me that all AAI had there were bookkeeping records, which they promptly sent to me. Ellen Walsh in White Plains said, "Oh, didn't you know, there was a fire at the AAI office and everything was destroyed." There was about $7,000 in our bank account, primarily from sales of our AAI directory and affiliation fees.

With almost no assets, I asked our Columbus pregnancy center executive director, in early spring of 1990, to allow AAI to open our administrative office in a large, walk-in closet at one of our client offices, on South James Road in Columbus. My husband and I had a big wooden desk (that I am currently writing on!) that had been given to us by a friend. We had that desk moved to the closet, I had a phone installed, and I bought a used, four-drawer, Steelcase file cabinet and a computer. That was the beginning of our Columbus Heartbeat International headquarters.

I also called Dr. John and Lore to tell them of the lack of records from Orlando and White Plains. To my shock and delight, Lore informed me that she had only sent copies of all the AAI materials to White Plains and she had, intact, all of the records from our founding through her resignation, plus

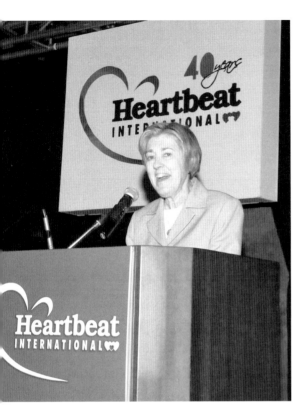

▲ *Sister Paula Vandegaer, one of Heartbeat International's three co-founders, is the first recipient of a new award, inaugurated at our Fortieth Anniversary Conference, the Heartbeat International Legacy Award, to honor people within Heartbeat International who have made an outstanding contribution to our movement that will be handed down to future generations.*

all the publications and board records up to that time! She and Dr. John invited me to come to Toledo to pick them up.

Although I didn't fully realize it at the time, this would be my last visit with our founders and my heroes and mentors, Dr. John and Lore. Dr. John had experienced a slight stroke. Although it was a quick blackout and he returned to normal, he was distraught that his physician had told him that he must retire from his medical practice and not risk another incident that could result in harm to one of his dear patients. Dr. John was eighty-two and quite upset—his medical practice was his life, and he complained that he had just signed a three-year phone system contract and was sure he couldn't get a refund!

In preparation for a move to live with his brother in another state, he was dismantling his large medical library, and he gave me one of his core textbooks on obstetrics and gynecology. (I recently found out that Dr. John's archives are now housed at Franciscan University in Steubenville, Ohio.) Lore presented me with several cartons of records, including all correspondence, many with notes and letters in her own handwriting, financial records, publications, and board minutes of AAI from the beginning. They helped me load the materials into the trunk of my car. What a treasure!

Dr. John, after moving to live with his brother, died in 1992. Although I talked to Lore several times by phone over the next several years and she was always supportive and encouraging, she was becoming very reclusive, focused on health and financial issues. She agreed to meet me for dinner in Toledo only one more time. She did not come in person for our Twenty-Fifth Anniversary celebration in 1996, at our Chicago conference, but she did send a congratulatory message that she read to me over the phone and that I delivered to the delegates.

We invited as many of that founding generation to our anniversary celebration as possible, and several were able to attend. To honor them, we inaugurated a special award called our Servant Leader Award, and gave it to these founders and longtime leaders. All of these heroes could lead effectively, build a team, and get results. Yet, each also had a great humility and modesty, and put others ahead of self.

When Heartbeat gives the Servant Leader awards now at each annual International Conference, we call to mind our role model, Jesus, the greatest of all servant leaders. Although He was Lord and God of all, He washed the feet of his disciples. And although He could have come down from the cross, He was obedient even to death in order to give His life in ransom for ours.

Lore eventually entered a hospice facility, suffering from cancer, in 2004. Esther Applegate, Dr. John's nurse, cared for her faithfully through her last years and planned her funeral. (Lore only had one living relative, her nephew, the son of the sister that she had been able to get out of Germany in 1945 to have her baby in safety.) I visited the funeral home, and Esther sent me a few of Lore's personal items, at my request.

Sister Paula, happily, is still actively working in our movement, traveling, teaching, and speaking. Not only did she found International Life Services in 1985, she continued a publication called *Living World* magazine for many years that contained articles on all areas of pro-life, from abortion to euthanasia. Her friend Kathy, who first dreamed and then sketched the picture of the girl in the forest, is still a key partner in Sister Paula's work. Sister also founded and directs a program called Volunteers for Life, a group of volunteers who live in community for one year and dedicate themselves to service agencies in the Los Angeles area. Sister wrote a textbook in 2000, *Introduction to Pregnancy Counseling*, with twelve supporting videos to teach counseling skills. Since 1967 she has been involved in the formation of more than one hundred pregnancy counseling centers, several of which are federated with her organization, and many are also affiliated with Heartbeat International.

I still consider her a dear partner and wise mentor, and Heartbeat International was honored to have her with us for our Fortieth Anniversary in 2011. We presented her with our first Legacy Award to honor her lasting contribution to Heartbeat International and to our movement.

A Call to Leadership and First Decisions

This chapter is the most personal of all in this first-forty-year history of the foot soldiers armed with love in the pregnancy help movement. It is the story of how I became the full-time leader of Heartbeat International. I am a little uncomfortable including such a personal story, but I decided to tell it because, having shared some of it in smaller groups, I know that many other Christians identify with it and have found it helpful.

It is the story of how a call can become so strong, and somewhat confusing, that you have to almost accept it "blindly" and trust entirely in the Lord, almost like when Jesus challenged His disciples to go further into the deep and cast their nets. I finally took this next step in my pro-life journey, and the Lord has never been unfaithful—He has rewarded me constantly with a deeper and deeper trust in Him and love for Him.

When I offered to become "acting chairman of the board" of AAI at that board meeting in Toledo in early 1990, when I was the only person left on the board to even consider assuming responsibility (see previous chapter), I thought that my job looked "doable": build up the board membership and find an executive director to lead the organization. I had served as chairman of the board of the local AAI affiliate in Columbus since my husband and I had helped found it (about ten years earlier), and, with a great working board team that became a great governing board, the organization had grown and developed, opened multiple office sites in the city, and hired excellent staff leadership. Becoming board chair of AAI seemed like a similar job.

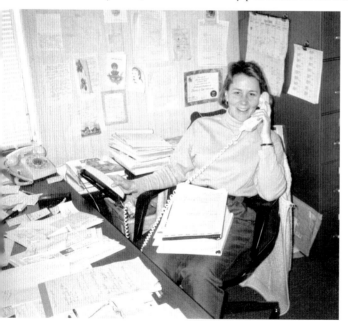

▲ *Peggy Hartshorn at her desk, with two phones, as the new president of Heartbeat International, 1994.*

In 1990, I was a professor of English at Franklin University in Columbus, Ohio, where I had begun teaching in 1974, right after I received my Ph.D. in English from The Ohio State University. I had interrupted full-time teaching in 1979 to stay home with our adopted son Tim and to have more time for my husband Mike. (On our Marriage Encounter weekend in 1978, the Lord convinced me that I was neglecting our marriage relationship, rushed as I was with Tim, teaching, and our volunteer pro-life work.) Although many on the faculty had told me I was wasting my education when I announced my resignation from the full-time faculty in 1979, one Christian professor, Don Collins, told me that he and his wife had prayed about it and were convinced that God would send us another child to adopt.

Later that same year, before I had even finished out my contract as a full-time professor, our daughter Katy was born. We were so fortunate to be able to adopt her. (Adoptions of infants in the United States had became very rare almost immediately after *Roe v. Wade* became the law of the land in 1973, with only 2–3 percent of single mothers making an adoption plan for their children. This is still true today.) This experience was one of many that the Lord has used, over the years, to show me that, when I follow His promptings, He provides in ways that put me in awe of Him.

I went back to full-time teaching at Franklin in 1987 when Katy was in third grade, Mike's and my relationship was strong, and the pregnancy center seemed to be humming along. I had wanted to be an English teacher since I was a little girl, so teaching at Franklin was a dream-come-true. As an English and humanities professor who read and commented on student journals and other writing daily, I thought I was also doing the Lord's work, since I could reinforce my students' religious beliefs and often provide a message of hope, all in a collegiate environment that was, from a national perspective, becoming more and more intolerant of Christians and critical of student expressions of Christianity in the classroom.

I soon was in charge of hiring all adjunct faculty who taught humanities and writing, and I developed several courses for the core curriculum. I felt I was influential in "holding the line" at Franklin and reinforcing a curriculum that, although multicultural, remained friendly to Western culture, with its roots not only in the classical era but also in Christianity. I had peer support on the faculty, and I belonged to a wonderful group of faculty members, Catholics, mainline Protestants, and Evangelical Christians, who prayed together and read and discussed a wide range of Christian books (including, for example, Francis A. Schaeffer's *How Should We Then Live?* and Thomas Aquinas's *Summa Theologica*). I loved my life as it was, seemingly just right.

As you might have guessed, I ran into more challenges than I could have imagined when I accepted the job as acting board chair of AAI, moved the administrative office to Columbus, and attempted to keep our core commitments to our affiliates. Several of the leaders I asked to serve on the AAI Board did not say "yes." It was difficult for the Columbus pregnancy center staff, which was helping with AAI business, to keep up with correspondence and other administrative functions. After the conference in Pittsburgh that was underway when I became acting chairman of the board, it proved almost impossible to find a host center for the next annual Academy. We finally organized a small Academy in Toledo, Ohio, for 1991. I was adamant that we would not interrupt our record of an Academy for affiliates every year since our founding in 1971.

I finally hired a part-time executive director for AAI, Andy Show, who had been the executive director of another nonprofit organization and was currently, along with his wife, a volunteer at our pregnancy center. Andy worked hard, but soon he got an opportunity to start a business. It proved so successful that he told me he could help us more as a donor, and he has been a major donor for Heartbeat, with a faithful annual pledge, ever since (nearly twenty years!).

I was feeling more and more guilty about accepting this responsibility but not being able to carry it out effectively. One letter that AAI received about that time affected me deeply. It was from a young Catholic lay missionary, a nurse named Judy Schell, who was in Eastern Europe. Somehow she had found AAI (this was before websites!), and she wrote us a letter, telling us about her work and asking for assistance to set up pregnancy centers in the Czech Republic. I knew that, based on AAI's mission, we should have been able to help, but I had to write her back and tell her that we had neither staff nor resources to provide help. I felt horrible. This motivated me to try even harder to get AAI back on its feet carrying out its crucial mission around the world.

I had found an affiliate to organize and provide hosting for our Academy for 1992, actually the strong coalition of pregnancy centers in Cincinnati, Ohio, one of the centers headed by an old friend of mine from high school, Patty Dannemiller. I had gotten to know the centers in this coalition, as well as their leader Mary Ann Boyd, and I was especially impressed with an Evangelical center headed by Carol Aronis.

It was our habit to have our annual board meeting at the same time and place as the Academy, and these were set for November 1992. I didn't realize that the board meeting was scheduled two days after the national presidential elections, but when we convened, Bill Clinton had just been elected president, to succeed George Bush, who had extended pro-life gains made originally under Reagan. I will never forget the "mood" of that meeting. It seemed that all the advances that the pro-life movement would now be lost forever.

This seemed confirmed by the fact that, earlier that same year, the Supreme Court had handed down a decision in *Planned Parenthood v. Casey*, a case originating in Pennsylvania, that was a tremendous disappointment. The Court upheld certain restrictions on abortion such as waiting periods, as long as they met a new standard invented by the Court: that they did not place an "undue burden" on the woman. Many had hoped that this case would end with a ruling that overturned *Roe v. Wade*, but, on a sharply divided court, it all depended on the vote of Supreme Court Justice Kennedy. Kennedy voted the other way, and the majority opinion stated, "No change in Roe's factual underpinning has left its central holding obsolete, and none supports an argument for its overruling."

At the time, it appeared that the political and legislative arms of the pro-life movement would be powerless, and that the only part of the movement that could save and change lives would be ours, the alternatives to abortion or service arm of the movement. The board and I felt an urgent call to step up to the plate. It seemed we had been gathered together for our meeting, two days after the election, for a reason—we were being called, like Esther, "for such a time as this."

Soon after the board meeting, I met Carol Aronis in the conference center. We moved away from the crowd and I stood next to a pillar. We discussed the current state of the nation and of our movement, and the fact that AAI was still, essentially, leaderless. Carol told me that she would follow me, and that she thought I was being called to lead AAI on a full-time basis. I remember falling back slightly against the pillar. I was conflicted at that point, but I didn't say anything. I was fighting with myself. I knew perhaps she was right, but I could not or did not want to believe it was true. My life was just the way I wanted it—if I could only pass on this burden of AAI to someone else!

From that time on, for over a year, I wrestled with myself and tried to discern what the Lord would have me do. My husband Mike was supportive, whatever I decided. We have always been committed to this work as a couple. I spoke to many Christians I knew, including our faculty discussion group at Franklin, my pastor, and other people whose spiritual insights I respected. One person gave me a book that contained a list of about ten ways that people discern what the Lord is calling them to do. I tried every one of the suggested processes, but still was conflicted. How could the Lord want me to give up the Christian mission I believed I had at Franklin, spend more time away from my husband and two teenaged children, give up the teaching that I loved, leave the board of the local center that I had helped found, and step into a full-time position as the leader of AAI?

Moreover, I was totally intimidated by the job and those who had gone before me. I was a teacher, not an administrator. Teaching had been my first and only job since college. Lore Maier had traveled all over the world and had contacts and friends on every continent, it seemed. She and her vision had driven our worldwide development. I had her box of correspondence with these internationals, dated from 1971 to 1982. Would those contacts still even be current? I had no idea how I could "tackle" the international aspect of our work. I had been to Europe, but that was the extent of my international travel. Dr. Hillabrand had hundreds, perhaps thousands, of medical contacts around the world. How could that be duplicated? Sister Paula was a professional social worker and counselor—I brought no credentials that were directly related to our work in pregnancy help centers. I was just an English teacher.

I made appointments with several consultants that various people referred me to—experts in organizational development and leadership. Although I bared my soul to these people, I somehow felt that they did not understand AAI and my situation, and they offered no real help. One kindly gentleman, seeing my distress, gave me the best piece of advice I got from these secular consultants. He ended our meeting by telling me that I probably could not duplicate or rebuild what our founders had built, and I probably should not take that as my task. The first relief I felt

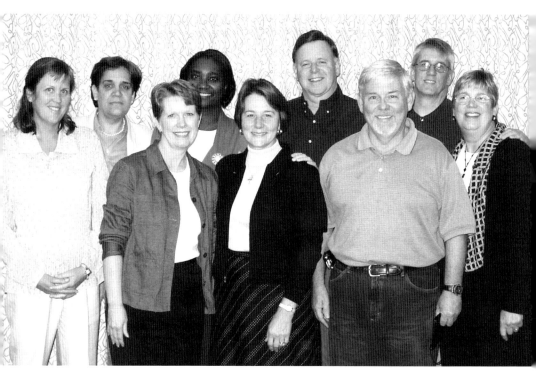

▲ *The Governing Board of Heartbeat International in 2004, with three "foundational board members" (Janet, Mike, and Anne) who served twelve years each on the board in our formative years. Pictured, back row, L to R: Mary Weyrick, Marry Suarez Hamm, Pat Hunter, Mike Hartshorn, Rev. John Ensor. Front row, L to R: Janet Trenda, Peggy Hartshorn, John Tabor, Anne Pierson.*

in this process of discernment came as a result of that meeting. If I was supposed to do this job, I had to walk in my own footsteps, so to speak.

Finally, one of the Evangelical Christians in our faculty discussion group, Tom Voight, who had told me that he saw a special "fire" in me when we prayed in our group about AAI, suggested that I might never know if I was supposed to take leadership of AAI on a full-time basis unless I tried it. He suggested I ask for a one-year leave of absence from Franklin University and try the job, and see how the Lord would lead me. That is what I did, in 1993.

Even during that first year when I threw myself into leading AAI on a daily basis, I was still conflicted about what I would do when my leave of absence was over. It was not until the moment after I handed my letter of resignation to the dean at Franklin, in spring of 1994, that I felt a gigantic load being lifted from my shoulders. I knew only then that I had made the right decision.

I still don't quite understand why it was so difficult for me to know what the Lord wanted me to do. At no other time in my life had I ever been unclear about the Lord's leading at a crucial time in my life. This experience, however, reinforced something that I have seen over and over again in my leadership of Heartbeat. Sometimes the Lord leads us to take a certain road, but He only lets us see clearly a few steps ahead. We need to trust Him that He will show us more clearly, as far as we need to see, as we go along. He always does this, thus building our trust in Him. To explain how I see this process, I have used the analogy of driving a car at night. The headlights let us see just enough ahead that we have confidence to keep moving at full speed. As we move, the road becomes clear, but only as far as we need to see it. (Sometimes, if it is foggy or rainy, that is not very far ahead, but we still keep cautiously moving!)

Once I submitted and said "yes" to whatever the Lord had in store for me, especially things outside my previous experience and skills, He began to show me that, indeed, He had prepared me for such a time as this. In fact, I know now that had I devoted myself full time to pro-life work, day in and day out, in those early years, right after *Roe v. Wade*, when sometimes I was passionate to do so, it would not have been good. I would not have been strong enough spiritually to withstand the attacks, and my relationship with Mike and my children would not have been strong enough either.

I will never forget my first few weeks on the job as "president." (I was uncomfortable with the title of executive director, perhaps because I had never been an executive!) I spent much of the time taking phone calls from our affiliates. They told me they needed a new training manual for volunteers and staff that were working with clients. I realized, I am a writer and teacher, with at least eighteen years experience working with pregnant girls, in our home, on our center's twenty-four-hour hotline, in our center offices, and I was taught by our founders. I have trained volunteers for years at our center in Columbus. A training manual is something I think I can do! Other affiliates asked for help with adoption programs and special cases. We had two adopted children, six of the twelve girls who lived in our home over the years made adoption plans for their children, and my husband Mike and I had walked with them every step of the way. I could help our affiliates with adoption issues and questions!

This kind of revelation continued. I saw that, indeed, God had prepared me for this job. I was in the right place at the right time for our affiliates. Even when situations occurred (and still do!) for which I had no previous experience to rely on, the Lord has always sent insights and wisdom, often through the people and partners He has sent to share the load: executive directors of our affiliated organizations, Heartbeat board members, advisors, benefactors, friends, family, and others!

In fact, three Heartbeat board members have served for twelve consecutive years since the early 1990s: my husband Mike, Anne Pierson, and Janet Trenda. (We now have a mandatory one-year leave after two three-year terms!) They and others have devoted uncountable hours, giving gifts of time, talent, and treasure, standing with me to help Heartbeat grow and develop. A list of Heartbeat International and AAI board members for our first forty years is in appendix III. These people have been core prayer partners, as well as discerning decision makers and "governors" for Heartbeat.

Besides committed board members, another blessing that the Lord has always provided for me is a wonderful staff, growing in number gradually through the years, from one to twenty-two at the present time (eleven full-time and eleven part-time). Each one has provided crucial gifts and skills.

Spiritual advisors have reminded me that Moses had Aaron, and he needed special helpers to hold up his arms so he could keep them outstretched while the army defeated the enemy. God has also provided me with daily working partners with whom I have been able to share all my joy, sorrows, and challenges. Beth Diemert was my key partner in leadership on the Heartbeat staff from 1995 to 2005, and Jor-El Godsey and Carla Cole now serve in that role. But the first key staff partner (and first employee of Heartbeat) was Judy Schell.

When I realized God was indeed calling me to become the full-time leader of Heartbeat, I remembered the nurse, Judy Schell, who had written me from Eastern Europe and asked for help. We had been corresponding, and I knew that she had just returned to the United States and was living with her parents in Pennsylvania. I could provide nothing at that time, but I called her and asked if she could partner with me so that we would never again have to turn down a request for help in starting pregnancy centers. She agreed to come to Columbus and be my "right hand" as long as we could pay her $1,000 per month to pay off her student loans. We agreed that she would live with Mike and me and our children, so she would have no additional living expenses.

One of our key decisions early on was to change our name from AAI to Heartbeat International. This was a difficult decision. "Alternatives to Abortion" had become the generic term in public use for the services we provided, like the corporate name Kleenex is commonly used as a generic name for tissue. The Yellow Pages, for example, used the headings "Alternatives to Abortion" to contrast with "Abortion Services." However, several people, including several experts in communications and public relations, had told me, "You need to get that word *abortion* out of your name. It polarizes people and has bad connotations." In fact, I experienced an adverse reaction when I had called hotels to ask for bids on our Academy in Cincinnati in 1992. The person in the sales office said, "Now, will the hotel need to prepare for public demonstrations or picketers?"

The board considered new names for over a year, but none of the suggestions seemed right. And how would people know that the new name was really us, AAI? Finally, I had a revelation and suggested that we take the name Heartbeat, a name that was not on our list but one that had been connected with us from our very first newsletter in 1972, and the name of our groundbreaking periodical *Heartbeat* magazine. I called Sister Paula and she had no objection. So, we became Heartbeat International officially.

Judy Schell and I developed the list of key services to be provided to affiliates from Heartbeat International, and we went about making sure we could provide them. We contacted the approximately 250 centers that had paid AAI $25 in any of the previous three years, for affiliation and a free AAI directory. Based on our new service plan and benefits, about 100 of those centers agreed to pay $100 for annual affiliation. They were the first official affiliates of Heartbeat

International. Judy became our first development director, fearlessly contacting potential donors by phone and letter and asking them to support our work. Thus we made sure that we could pay her salary of $1,000 per month and our basic expenses. I became a salaried employee about three years later.

Meanwhile, I looked for excellent training and program manuals that had been developed by our affiliates, and asked for permission to publish and distribute some of them more widely as "Model Program Manuals." Out of that came our abortion recovery manual called *H.E.A.R.T.* (Healing the Effects of Abortion Related Trauma) from Pregnancy Distress Center in Columbus, and our *Bridges Manual* from Alternate Avenues in California (a version of the now popular "Earn While You Learn" program, published later by Dinah Monahan, a Heartbeat affiliate whose family owns Heritage House '76, and whose mother developed the little feet pin). Thus our affiliates could help each other in a spirit of collegiality.

I looked for a general volunteer "counselor" training manual that would meet the needs of our diverse group of affiliates, but did not find one. I met two other leaders in our movement who were working on training manuals, but they did not have a vision for writing a manual that would meet the needs of both Catholic and Evangelical volunteer "counselors" (who filled the USA centers) as well as counselors in other countries, some with radically different cultures. So, I also started working on the new training manual that many of our affiliates had requested. I had been training the volunteers and staff at our local pregnancy center, Pregnancy Distress Center (now Pregnancy Decision Health Centers), and other centers in central Ohio. The system I had developed over that ten-year period finally became *The LOVE Approach*™, first edition published in 1994 (updated in 2005, with a new edition in 2011). *The LOVE Approach* has become the signature piece for Heartbeat International and will be discussed more fully in the next chapter.

When I said yes to leadership of Heartbeat International twenty years ago, I never would have imagined what the Lord had in store for this foot soldier. If you have not already joined His army, do so, and be amazed at how He will use you too!

A Christ-Centered Army

The most important early decision I made as the president of Heartbeat International was to describe Heartbeat explicitly as a Christian organization. Heartbeat had always been composed of Christian people—it was a movement of the church, the Body of Christ. But the terms used to describe it up to this point, "nondenominational and nonsectarian," had led to a variety of interpretations from affiliates. These ranged from "I guess we can describe ourselves as a Christian ministry, but not a Baptist, or Catholic, or Presbyterian one," to "We cannot have anything in our center or our programs that would hint that we are Christians—it might turn away clients or make them believe we are forcing our views on them."

I struggled with the decision to call Heartbeat International a Christian organization, not because I was unsure if it was the right decision—I had no doubt that it was. But I struggled because I did not know how it would be accepted among our affiliates and what unforeseen consequences it might bring.

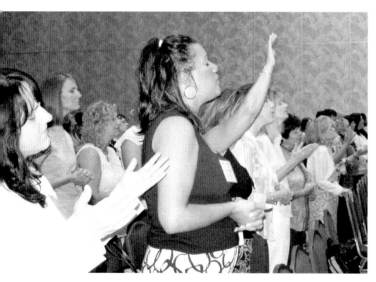

▲ Daily praise and worship opportunities, daily Mass, and individual prayer times are very much appreciated by participants at the Heartbeat International Conference, no matter what expression of Christianity they profess. They often share that our conferences and other training opportunities provide nourishment for the spirit, as well as for the mind and heart.

AAI was, from the beginning, an outreach of and by Christian people. (There was only one non-Christian woman I ever met within Heartbeat, and she headed an agency that was staffed primarily by Catholics.) In a talk given at our Twenty-Fifth Anniversary Conference in 1996, Sister Paula used the term "first wave" to describe the Catholics who had been the predominant force in the early years of the pro-life movement, and the term "second wave" to describe the Evangelical Christians and other Protestants

Protestants who began to enter the movement in the late seventies and early eighties, motivated in large part by Francis Schaeffer and Dr. C. Everett Koop. They toured the country in 1979, showing the galvanizing pro-life film *Whatever Happened to the Human Race.*

One of the effects of this influx of the "second wave" was that centers with an explicitly Evangelical statement of faith were intentionally developed by the new organization called Christian Action Council (their first center opening in Baltimore in 1981), with support from Catholics and AAI (see chapter 5). Another effect was that Evangelical Christians were volunteering in large numbers in some of the original AAI centers. This had happened at the center I helped found, Pregnancy Distress Center, in Columbus, Ohio. During our very first week of operation, we welcomed many Evangelical Christians as volunteers who had seen press coverage of our grand opening on January 22, 1981. So, when I became president of Heartbeat, I had personally worked closely with both Catholics and Evangelicals at our center for ten years, and I loved it. There were always challenges, but solving the issues as they arose brought great rewards. It was a blessing that our center had the support of a large number of both Catholic and Protestant churches and a broad base of community support.

Working with other strong Christians deepened my own faith and gave me a new passion for evangelism. It prompted me to read what the Catholic Church taught about evangelism, and I was moved greatly by John Paul II's encyclical, issued in 1990, Mission of the Redeemer (*Redemptoris Missio*), in which he wrote, "Every person has a right to hear the 'Good News.'"

I also came across the eloquent and inspirational document "Evangelicals and Catholics Together," initiated by Chuck Colson of Prison Fellow Ministries and Father Richard John Neuhaus of the Institute on Religion and Public Life, and signed onto by thirty-nine scholars and Christian leaders including Rev. Pat Robertson, Dr. Richard Land, Dr. Bill Bright, Dr. Os Guinness, Rev. Avery Dulles, John Cardinal O'Connor, George Weigel, and Michael Novak. It was published on March 29, 1994. (Over the years, they issued other joint statements worthy of note.)

The authors made a clear list of the core Christian beliefs on which Evangelicals and Catholics agree, and a list of those issues (doctrine, worship, practice, and piety) where we "continue to search together—through study, discussion, and prayer—for a better understanding of one another's convictions and a more adequate comprehension of the truth of God in Christ." They then urged strong Christians to work together, or "contend together," in the modern world that so opposes Christ. The statement specifically discussed the importance of Evangelicals and Catholics working together on the issue of abortion, calling abortion "the leading edge of an encroaching culture of death." It commends the pregnancy help center movement specifically and our efforts for the sake of the unborn, mothers, and fathers.

Its conclusion I still find inspiring. It matched then (and still does now) my passion for Christians to work together in the hostile world in which we live, transcending our theological differences, in order to most effectively carry out the our mission:

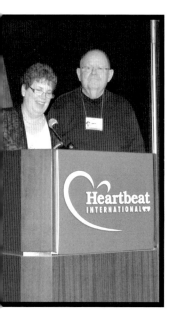

We do not know, we cannot know, what the Lord of history has in store for the third millennium. It may be the springtime of world missions and great Christian expansion. It may be the way of the cross, marked by persecution and apparent marginalization. In different places and times, it will likely be both. Or it may be that Our Lord will return tomorrow. We do know that His promise is sure, that we are enlisted for the duration, and that we are in this together. We do know that we must affirm and hope and search and contend and witness together, for we belong not to ourselves but to Him who has purchased us by the blood of the cross. We do know that this is a time of opportunity—and, if of opportunity, then of responsibility— for Evangelicals and Catholics to be Christians together in a way that helps prepare the world for the coming of Him to whom belongs the kingdom, the power, and the glory forever. Amen.

▲ *Anne and Jimmy Pierson, founders of House of His Creation maternity home and the international ministry Loving and Caring, were honored with one of the inaugural Legacy Awards at Heartbeat's Fortieth Anniversary International Conference. They were instrumental, beginning in the AAI years, in focusing the pregnancy help movement on our opportunities for Christian ministry, especially as our affiliates become involved one-on-one with mentoring of the mothers and fathers whom the Lord sends to us.*

One of my most faith-filled colleagues in the movement was (and is) Anne Pierson, a strong Evangelical Christian, whom I first met when she was a presenter at AAI Academies. She and her husband, Jimmy, were a great inspiration to me and other attendees. They began housing pregnant girls in their own home in the 1970s, eventually founding a maternity home called House of His Creation. It was definitely faith-based, and Anne and Jimmy shared openly at the AAI Academies about evangelizing these women by pouring into them and reflecting to them the love of Jesus day by day. They pioneered a new kind of maternity home (to replace the large institutional home common in the 1950s and 1960s before the Supreme Court decision *Roe v. Wade* in 1973), a home of father, mother, and children that also welcomed pregnant girls and women and modeled with them the family as God intended.

Anne and Jimmy not only witnessed to us on a gentle and loving evangelism, they also spoke into our movement the values of fatherhood and adoption. Over the years, Anne and Jimmy lived with two hundred girls, and about one hundred of them made adoption plans for their babies. Anne and Jimmy are still in contact with most of these women, a demonstration of their true love for these children of God.

I always admired Anne and Jimmy tremendously, and Anne was one of the first people I asked to serve in leadership as a member of the Heartbeat International Board. She did so for twelve consecutive years, in our most formative time. In recognition of this tremendous legacy that Anne and Jimmy have given our movement, Heartbeat awarded them our Legacy Award during our fortieth anniversary year.

At one of our early board meetings, I believe it was Anne's suggestion that we write down what we think God is going to do through the new Heartbeat International. We all agreed on the first item: He would use Heartbeat International to continue to bring together the church, the Body of Christ, especially bringing together Catholics and Protestants. The Lord has now been doing this mightily through Heartbeat, and I and our present board and staff are totally committed to continue to allow the Lord to work through us to this end.

We celebrate our unity in diversity on our board, always intentionally trying to keep a balance between Catholics and Protestants in our numbers. We have various board members leading us in prayer, and we enjoy our different styles and approaches in praying to and worshipping the Lord. Sometimes we informally discuss our theological differences and try to understand them better, and often we discover that we agree more than we disagree. We find those discussions to be challenging and faith building.

As we developed the new Heartbeat International, beginning in 1993, I wanted it to be clear that we were still the "big umbrella" envisioned by our founders in the early 1970s that welcomed many models and forms of pregnancy help ministries. They could be primarily composed of Catholics, or of Evangelicals, or of Orthodox Christians, or they could be mixed. They could have a purpose of explicitly *sharing* Christ with clients, as some did, or they could see their role primarily as *being* Christ to their clients through serving them in their hour of need, as some did.

They could be inspired and led by the Biblical command "Go into all the world and preach the good news to all creation"(Mark 16:15, NIV), as many of the "second wave" centers were. Or, they could be inspired by the Biblical command, "I assure you, as often as you did it for one of my least brothers, you did it for me" (Matt. 25:40, NAB), as many of the "first wave" centers were. They could have an explicit, formal "Statement of Faith" for volunteers, board, and staff to sign, or they could not have one. Some centers at that time had a statement of faith adapted from the National Council of Evangelicals, some had adopted the Apostles' Creed or Nicene Creed, and some had developed a statement of faith through discussions among Christians of various denominations who were working in their center.

Since our founding in 1971, the culture had dramatically changed, and client needs had changed too. Then, it could be presumed that the culture was basically a Judeo-Christian one and that this would be reflected in most community-based organizations. For example, my husband was president of the Columbus Big Brother Association in the 1970s. Their community events always started with a prayer, and speakers routinely talked about their relationship with the Lord when they described their motivation to become Big Brothers. By the 1990s, however, this was no longer to be expected. Charitable organizations were distancing themselves from explicit Christianity. It was becoming "politically incorrect" to make one's Christianity public.

When I became president in 1993, some centers that inquired about affiliation wanted to be sure that all our training materials and programs would be Biblically based. I needed to assure them that they would, indeed. At that point also, abortion recovery programs were becoming more and more essential in our work, if we were to truly serve the women the Lord was sending us both as clients and volunteers. How could we have an effective program that did not explicitly focus on the forgiveness available from our Lord?

So, I described Heartbeat International in 1993 as "an interdenominational Christian association" of life-affirming service providers, and dropped "nondenominational and nonsectarian" from our vocabulary. I announced this explicitly in our newsletter, and I did not receive even one objection from our affiliates. Rather, I received several calls and letters thanking me for making it clear that Heartbeat is a Christian organization.

I was not then, and am not now, totally happy with the word choice since many churches do not see themselves as "denominations," and sometimes the term "Christian" is thought to refer to primarily "born again Christian," and some do not think of it as including Catholic Christians (this was especially true in 1993). The term "ecumenical" did not seem a good one then, since to many Catholics at the time the term connoted something that was "lukewarm." (Recently, the term "ecumenical" is beginning to have more positive connotations!)

Today, we refer to Heartbeat as a "Christ-centered association" of life-affirming service providers. Heartbeat's core values statement cites the Nicene Creed as an expression of the core beliefs that unify all Christians. We are the "big umbrella" that I described earlier, and our affiliates have autonomy in how they handle this issue within their own organizations.

Our explicit, Christ-centered orientation would be demonstrated in the first and core training manual of Heartbeat, published in 1994, *Planting the Seed: The LOVE Approach*, now called simply *The LOVE Approach Training Manual*™. Clearly Biblically based, it takes its inspiration from the parable of the sower in Matthew 13:3–8, and from chapter 13 of St. Paul's first letter to the Corinthians, sometimes called St. Paul's hymn to love.

Taking my inspiration from Sister Paula's training, I first focused, in *The LOVE Approach*, on developing a personal relationship with the client, listening to her, and affirming her dignity as a person. I added things my husband Mike and I had learned through couples communication courses (in conjunction with our Marriage Encounter), such as the Awareness Wheel that focuses on listening to the other person's thoughts, feelings, wants, values, and beliefs. I knew that sometimes Mike and I had been able, using the Awareness Wheel, to sort through difficult problems and issues and make a decision that fit within our values and beliefs. This became the L step, Listen and Learn, of *The LOVE Approach*.

Being a teacher, I added a component to the process that is educational and informational to help the person understand all her possible choices, presented in a loving and caring way that avoids debating or arguing with a client. In the case of the pregnant client, her options are either abortion or parenting through one of three options: adoption, single parenting, or marriage. In the case of the non-pregnant client, they are sexual promiscuity or sexual integrity. This became the O step, Open Options.

Having become convinced during my own experience with clients that we must "always be ready to explain the hope we have" and "do this with gentleness and respect" (1 Peter 3:15, NIV), I added an opportunity to share with our clients explicitly that they are special and valuable. They are made in the Image of God, and they are loved so much that God became man to redeem them with His blood. Regardless of what they have done, they can be forgiven and have a relationship with the God, through Jesus, who made and loves them so much. This became the V step, Vision and Value.

Another of our roles is to provide practical help and ongoing support to our clients as they carry through their positive life choices. This became the E step, Extend and Empower.

LOVE is not only the acronym for the steps of our process, but it is the source: love comes from God, God is love, and we reflect Him to the people He sends to us. We do this through who we are (as long as we remain in relationship with Him) and through what we do and say. Thus, we can both BE Christ to our clients and well as explicitly SHARE Christ with our clients, as led by the Holy Spirit. I acknowledge in *The LOVE Approach* that different ministries have different policies and teachings about how and when the Gospel is to be shared. Love is also the method of our approach to the client, as in St. Paul's description:

> *If I speak with human tongues and angelic as well, but do not have love, I am a noisy gong, a clanging cymbal. If I have the gift of prophecy and, with full knowledge, comprehend all mysteries, if I have faith great enough to move mountains, but have not love, I am nothing. If I give everything I have to feed the poor and hand over my body to be burned, but have not love, I gain nothing. Love is patient; love is kind. Love is not jealous, it does not put on airs, it is not snobbish. Love is never rude, it is not self-seeking, it is not prone to anger; neither does it brood over injuries. Love does not rejoice in what is wrong but rejoices with the truth. There is no limit to love's forbearance, to its trust, its hope, its power to endure. Love never fails. (I Cor. 13:1–8, NAB)*

I truly believe that *The LOVE Approach* was an inspiration from the Lord. It has stood the test of time (an updated edition was published in 2005 and again in 2011, our fortieth anniversary year), and it has been adapted for all kinds of service models now in existence in our movement (counseling, medical, residential, adoption agency, abortion recovery, and more). It has also been proven to be culturally adaptable and universal in many ways. It is used in centers that have primarily Protestant or Catholic staff and volunteers, in those that are denominational, such as Baptist centers, or in those that are mixed. It is used well in cities, small towns, and rural areas, for all ethnic groups. It is widely used around the world, and Heartbeat has provided special licenses for use in Africa, Asia, Latin America, and Australia. It is the first training course to become available online through the new Heartbeat Academy (named in honor of the first AAI Academies).

The LOVE Approach is also a method that can and should be used with family and friends, and with staff and board, indeed, with all those that we are in a relationship with, as we grapple through options with each other in any particular situation.

Moreover, the four steps of *The LOVE Approach* can be used by every person who encounters another person with an unexpected pregnancy. Women who are unsure about their options and who are vulnerable to abortion are in our own families, at our work places, in our churches and neighborhoods; they may be friends on Facebook or in our social network. Thus, every person reading this manual can become a foot soldier armed with LOVE and save and change lives! *The LOVE Approach* outline can be downloaded from the Heartbeat International website, and a more detailed training is available online through Heartbeat.

Our first major change, to reflect our new Christian identity, was in our annual conference. At the 1994 conference in Columbus, Ohio, to our full program of general sessions and workshops, we added an interdenominational prayer service. In 1995, at the Pittsburgh conference, we added a daily time of praise and worship, and that has been a part of our conferences ever since. Most often we had an Evangelical worship team, but I remember when we were in Pittsburgh again, in 2002, and we could invite a praise and worship team from Franciscan University in Steubenville, a nearby Catholic college. I expected that the participants would not notice the "difference"—and I was right!

After the first couple of years of great praise and worship sessions, Catholic attendees asked if we might consider adding early morning Mass at the hotel, which we did. A few years later, they requested a special time available for Confessions. Would our Protestant brothers and sisters accept these changes, we wondered? They did. After many years, these options have become the expectation, and more and more people who attend our conferences, both Protestants and Catholics, comment positively on the spiritual "wealth" available. It's hard to believe that at one time we feared these changes might fatally disrupt our hard-fought unity. The devil would have loved to create disunity and harm our movement, but the Lord protected us.

In 2000, I attended a retreat weekend for the foot soldiers in our movement, sponsored by an Evangelical organization called "Second Question," that included Charismatic prayer teams that were available to pray over participants. I was moved to invite these prayer teams to provide optional individual prayer at our next annual conference, and to bring a team of intercessors to pray for us throughout the conference. I did this because our army seemed more and more to be under attack. There was great "woundedness" in our ranks, from abortions, broken marriages, disrupted relationships with children, attacks within the pregnancy help centers themselves, and competition and disunity among centers and among some national organizations in the pregnancy help movement. I saw the healing and restoration that had taken place at the retreat, and I believed the Lord wanted me to provide an opportunity for participants at our next conference. I discussed and prayed seriously about this with the leader of our affiliate services, Beth Diemert.

This was very risky. Many Catholics and Protestants are skeptical of Charismatics. How would opportunity for prayer and healing be accepted? Was I truly listening to the Lord? I decided to go forward with the plan for our next conference. It was in Glendale, California. The conference took place only two weeks after September 11, 2001. As it happened, we could not have picked a more opportune time to devote so much of our conference to prayer.

I remember being very anxious before the conference started, and the prayer teams prayed over me. I had invited every one of the leaders of all the national organizations in our movement to be part of a session of prayer to start the conference. Almost every one of these national leaders came and prayed publicly in their own way—Baptist, Catholic, Reformed, Nondenominational, Lutheran, Pentecostal, and more! The individual prayer times at that conference, and succeeding ones, went beautifully, and we still today have opportunities for individuals to come for personal prayer with a prayer team at our conference. Diverse prayer and worship opportunities are now such a natural and accepted part of who Heartbeat is, and what our affiliates appreciate, that it is hard to imagine how much courage, on the part of the Heartbeat leadership team, it took to provide these opportunities the first time around.

Our centers have a wide variety of ways of sharing the Gospel within their centers. Heartbeat suggests gentle ways of introducing the Good News in *The LOVE Approach*, our core resource for affiliates. We also train centers to use the Biblically based *Peacemakers* program to help resolve conflict in their board, staff, and personal relationships within the centers. We teach centers in our *DIRECT Well*™ and *GOVERN Well*™ trainings (for directors and boards) that we must always follow high standards as promulgated in the professions that relate to our work: counseling, medical, accounting, fundraising, business, and others. But we must also "sift out" anything that contradicts basic Christian ethics.

Heartbeat tries to model Christ-like behavior in all we say and do, and in all our relationships with our affiliates and with other national and international organizations. We believe the Lord is using Heartbeat International in a mighty way to help create a Culture of Life around the world, and this means more than reducing the number of abortions. It means reflecting clearly, in every way we can, the love of Jesus, in our thoughts, words, and deeds.

Heartbeat and probably the majority of our affiliates were incorporated for "charitable purposes" when they became nonprofit organizations in their states and when they applied to the IRS for a status that would allow gifts to be tax-deductible. The IRS gives this coveted status (501c3) to organizations that can show charitable, religious, and/or educational purposes. Heartbeat eventually amended our articles of incorporation and notified the IRS that we have added "religious purposes" to "charitable purposes." And we advise that our affiliates consider the same. This gives us the most protection possible in asserting our right to be exempt from federal, state, and local laws that prohibit discrimination in hiring on the basis of religion and sexual orientation. We are prepared to defend our right to be a faith-based, nonprofit organization that lives out the Biblically based values that are at the core of our visions, mission, and programs.

Steering the Movement Into Areas of Greatest Need

One or our major challenges in this battle for the sanctity of human life, this epic struggle to save the most innocent and vulnerable among us and their mothers from abortion, is that the prime battlegrounds, the abortion clinics, are most often located in the areas where the army, the foot soldiers armed with love, are most in need of reinforcements, training, encouragement, and even new battle plans. In the United States, most abortions are performed in the heart of our major cities (our "NFL cities"). Most pregnancy centers, however, are located in mid-sized cities, small towns, and rural areas.

Heartbeat realized this early on. One of our early outreaches after I became president in 1993 was to schedule a series of "Regional Conferences" around the country. We wanted to meet the foot soldiers in our army, find out more about their needs and what they were doing, and bring Heartbeat resources to them. We used our *Worldwide Directory*, which listed all the United States centers by state, to send invitations to the leaders when we were going to be in their region.

Once we got to the northeastern states, we realized that there was a glaring problem. A vast number of abortions were being performed in that region of the country, but there was a very small number of pregnancy centers. From a cursory look, it appeared that two major problem areas were Boston and New York City, where numerous abortion clinics were located but only a handful of pregnancy centers.

In 1993 or 1994, my husband and I were in Boston, and as was my habit, I looked in the Yellow Pages to see how many abortion clinics there were and how many pregnancy centers. I called one of only two pregnancy centers (there were many abortion providers advertised), introduced myself as the president of Heartbeat International, and asked if I could come by to see the center. What I found was a very small office where the dedicated founder of this new center, a Baptist minister named John Ensor, was the only person present. He was there to answer the phone and see clients. He welcomed me warmly, and we shared our visions—his to make a difference for life in Boston, plagued with several abortion clinics, and mine to help centers like his make a difference for life throughout the United States and around the world.

That one small center in Boston, under John's leadership and in partnership with Heartbeat, grew to become the first pregnancy help medical clinic in the country with a physician as a paid staff member. Called A Woman's Concern, it grew to six offices (one on Cape Cod), while, at the same time, six abortion businesses closed. Thousands of Christians in the Boston area, Catholic

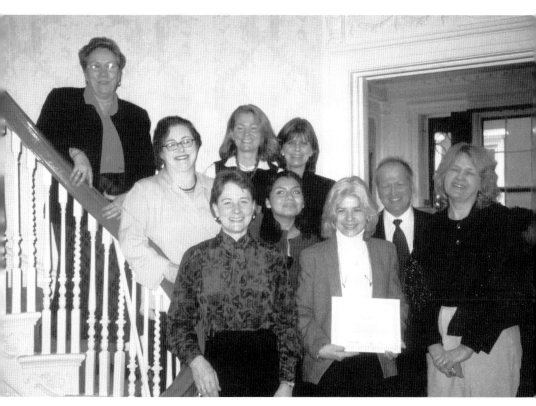

▲ *One of the many Heartbeat Project REACH trainings for directors, staff, board members, and volunteers in the New York City area from 1999 to the present. This was the first national "urban initiative" to bring attention to the fact that major urban areas in the United States have large numbers of abortion clinics and often only a few, heroic pregnancy help centers that need special support. Pictured, L to R: Loraine Gariboldi (Life Center of Long Island), Kathleen Elder (Boro Pregnancy Counseling Center), Peggy Hartshorn, Angela McNaughton (Pregnancy Care Center Inc.), Ellen Gavin, Dr. Elaine Eng (Boro Pregnancy Counseling Center), Linda Marzula (EMC Pregnancy Center), John Margand (executive director, Project REACH), Arlene Schroer (Northport Care Center). Linda is receiving her certificate as the first graduate of Heartbeat's ConCert program, the first distance-learning program for pregnancy center staff, initiated through Project REACH.*

and Protestant, joined the battle, as volunteers, staff, and board members, prayer partners, and financial partners who pledged $1.00 per day (the cost of a cup of coffee at that time!) to help this ministry grow and develop. Eventually, it was sophisticated enough to apply for and receive several federal and state grants for abstinence education programs in the Boston schools.

Heartbeat International knew that what was being accomplished in Boston through the Body of Christ and power of the Lord needed to be accomplished in other major American cities. In 1996,

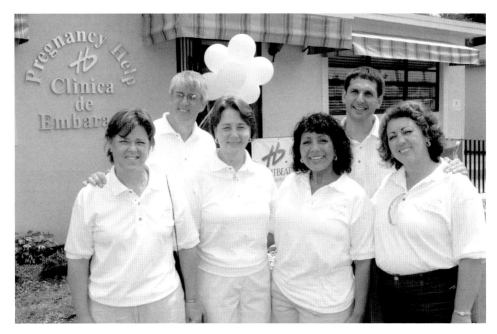

▲ *Urban Initiatives Executive Director John Ensor and his wife Kristen (first and second from left) moved to Miami for two years to awaken the Christian community there to the need for pregnancy help medical clinics. (Miami had thirty-seven abortion clinics.) They are pictured at the opening of Heartbeat of Miami's Hialeah clinic in 2007. Also pictured, L to R, are Peggy Hartshorn and the first staff members of Heartbeat of Miami, Martha Avila, David Behar, and Jeannie Pernia.*

Heartbeat developed what we called the "East Coast Project," later "Project Salt and Light," and began to seek funding for specific center development in the northeast. I had a heart especially for New York City. I had met one of the dedicated soldiers there, Chris Slattery, and I knew that there were about one hundred known abortion providers in the city at that time (including clinics, hospitals, and private doctors who advertised abortions) and only a handful of small pregnancy help centers, none of them with ultrasound services. Maybe the Lord could use Heartbeat to help.

I decided to call all of the centers in the New York City area that were listed in our *Worldwide Directory*, and see if I could arrange a small gathering to let them know about Heartbeat. As I look back, I realize that Heartbeat's initial offer of help (training, manuals, consultation, advice, networking, and prayer support) doesn't sound like much, considering the fact that New York City performed then (and still does) about one-fourth of all the abortions done in the United States and is sometimes called the "abortion capital" of the United States.

But God worked in mighty ways and used our first attempt there to inspire not only great work in New York City but also around the country through what came to be called, in our movement, the "Urban Initiatives." These were and are efforts to bring a Culture of Life into our cities, led by the people of those cities, especially African Americans and Latinos. It is one of the greatest examples in recent history of the church rising up to battle the forces of evil, armed with love. But let's see how it all got started in New York City.

As I started to call the existing pregnancy help centers in New York City to arrange an exploratory meeting, I realized the centers did not even know each other. Some center directors, fearful of attack from pro-abortion opponents, kept their home phone numbers secret (even from their office staff and volunteers), so it was very difficult to contact everyone. Finally, one of the center directors offered to have the gathering at her parish church, and we set a date. I made my plane reservations, the most reasonable being into Newark, New Jersey.

In every other city or town I had visited to do training or work with the center in some way, the director was eager to pick me up at the airport and offered to host me in her home (to save costs). No one mentioned that in New York City. I found out I could get a bus from New Jersey to the Grand Central Station area for about $10. Not willing or able to pay New York hotel costs, I was able to get a list of religious houses in major U.S. cities that would accept "pilgrims." The only one in New York City that had an opening was an old brownstone in the Greenwich Village area. It had one room available (shared bath down the hall) for the first night of my stay, but the second night all the rooms were full. They mentioned I could move into the pastor's office, which had a futon, for night two, since he didn't use his office on the weekend. The cost was a donation, suggested at $40 a night. I booked it.

My New York adventure of faith had begun, and that faith was dramatically rewarded!

At that first meeting, September 25, 1997, graciously arranged at Immaculate Conception Church on East 14th Street in New York City by Barbara Prado (from Life Center in Brooklyn), the following centers were represented: Pregnancy Care Center in New Rochelle; Good Counsel Homes on Staten Island; A Woman's Concern in Red Bank, New Jersey; Expectant Mother Care in New York City; Crossroad Pregnancy Resource Center on Staten Island; Life Center in Brooklyn; Pregnancy Help in New York City; and Bridge to Life in Bayside. Most representatives there did not know each other well, if at all. They had no coalition (common in other cities and regions).

In our frank and honest meeting, I began to understand how difficult it was to do our work in New York City, and how much courage and stamina these foot soldiers had. Some centers indicated that their staff and volunteers had to commute over an hour to get to the centers, cost of office rental space was exorbitant, advertising in the Yellow Pages was so costly that only a couple of the centers had one-line ads amidst the pages of large abortion clinic ads. Most importantly, the work was difficult and exhausting, with almost every client abortion-minded. New York paid for abortions, so it was the primary option that almost every woman considered.

The existing centers were understaffed and underfunded. The churches seemed almost oblivious to their situation and need. Very few Evangelical churches were supporting two small centers, one in Manhattan, and one on Long Island. The famous and beloved pro-life hero, Cardinal John J. O'Connor of New York City, had proclaimed that any woman who needed help with a crisis pregnancy could come to the church, so many Catholics presumed that the need for alternatives to abortion was met. However, that was not at all the case. Abortion percentages were very high in all the boroughs, with about half of all pregnancies ending in abortion in Brooklyn.

The centers present welcomed the help of Heartbeat International. That was the beginning of many memorable trips over several years to New York City for me and several members of the Heartbeat International team, which included Beth Diemert, who directed all our affiliate services, Rev. John Ensor, who came from Boston to provide help, and Carol Aronis, another Heartbeat consultant from Cincinnati, the person who had called me into Heartbeat leadership. On my second trip, how different things were. The director of Pregnancy Help, Anne Manice, hosted me in her home in Manhattan and introduced me to one of her board members, Bill Powers, who was especially interested in our project to help New York City.

We eventually named it Project REACH. The acronym means: R—Reach those at Risk for abortion; E—Educate them about their options; A—Advertise abortion alternative services; C—Develop Centers to strengthen their services and foundations; and H—Add Health and Healing services, especially ultrasound to save more lives and post-abortion recovery programs to reduce repeat abortions (because 50 percent of all abortions are abortions performed on someone who has already had one but has not been healed).

Bill Powers invited me, on my third visit to New York City, to his exclusive club near Central Park to introduce me to a friend of his whom he thought would also have an interest in the project. Bill's friend (who prefers to remain anonymous) told me that he had just sold his business and, for the first time in many years, he had the time to get involved in something other than his business that he cared deeply about, pro-life. He got involved wholeheartedly, donating space in his midtown Manhattan townhouse (that had been his office hub) for a Project REACH office and training center, and providing major funding for the project, pledged over five years. This was the largest gift Heartbeat had ever received up to that point. That a person of such influence and business acumen had the confidence in Heartbeat International to invest in such a major way in our project was a turning point for us. It was both a humbling and confidence-building experience.

In 1997, we hired Mary Kate Kelly (daughter of pro-life and abstinence pioneer Molly Kelly) to be our local liaison, and she set up an office in the townhouse, commuting from Philadelphia weekly. We conducted bimonthly trainings for all the centers, bringing in experts in various fields of organizational growth and development. We provided training in *The LOVE Approach* and abortion recovery so center programs could be strengthened.

We were able to get every New York City center (fourteen locations, ten organizations) to participate in a joint advertising campaign, and we took out a full-page ad in every New York

City Yellow Pages Directory, putting them in competition, for the first time, with the New York City abortion clinics. Because the subject heading Abortion Alternatives came before Abortion Services, our centers were listed in front of every abortion clinic in the city.

Project REACH also funded the first-ever distance learning program in our movement, the ConCert (Consultant Certificate) program of Heartbeat International, basically an adult-education, college-level course in pregnancy center counseling. Many of the New York City pregnancy center consultants (volunteer and staff) were trained in the program, and the first proud graduate was Linda Marzula from Expectant Mother Care.

Eventually, we hired an attorney, John Margand, to head up the project. He later applied for and received a federal grant for Project REACH that funded the first abstinence education program to be provided in New York City schools, called Healthy Respect. Federal grants are continuing to fund abstinence education in the Yonkers school district through Project REACH. John just retired from the project in 2010, and it is now headed by Dr. Nanci Coppola.

The pregnancy centers in New York City still face major hurdles, but progress has been made. Some centers provide ultrasound through contracts with private physicians. There is now a strong coalition of pregnancy help centers that meets regularly, and the leaders help and support each other. They are no longer alone. (New York City centers have recently been under attack with restrictive regulations passed by the New York City Council. This will be discussed more fully in chapter 11.)

In 2004, Heartbeat decided to find out what other parts of the country had too many abortion clinics and too few pregnancy help centers. Using the limited technology available, websites, online Yellow Pages, and a MapQuest-type system including most of the pregnancy help centers in the country, we developed a list of all of the abortion clinics in the United States, city by city, and then listed the closest center(s), indicating how many miles they were from the abortion clinics. It was very revealing, showing that many clusters of abortion clinics have only one or two pregnancy help centers nearby, and some of the clinics did not have a pregnancy center within twenty miles or more!

I took this study to a meeting of all of the pregnancy help center organization leadership (called the National Leadership Alliance, to be discussed in chapter 10), and they seemed stunned by the findings. It was clear that, up to this time, we had been trying to keep up with the growth of our movement wherever it was occurring, as the Holy Spirit was raising up people around the world to do this Great Work. But now we needed to be strategic and intentional in helping to steer our movement into areas of greatest need—to go into our major cities, where there were few, if any, pregnancy help centers, and "wake up" the churches to start them!

It was also clear that abortion clinics were disproportionately located in African American and Latino neighborhoods, and abortion providers were targeting other immigrant neighborhoods as well. In fact, even today the African American and Latino populations combined are only about 24 percent of the population, but over 50 percent of all abortions are performed on Latinos and African Americans.

Other organizations got into the effort. Focus on the Family, then headed by Dr. James Dobson in Colorado Springs, already had a department to help pregnancy centers. They held a series of meetings to discuss the shocking disparity between abortion clinics and pregnancy centers in metropolitan areas, and called the discussions "Impacting High Abortion Communities." Care Net was Heartbeat's partner in Option Line (see chapter 10). The president of Care Net, Kurt Entsminger, and I agreed to institute projects that we would both call "Urban Initiatives," and we would choose key cities where we would each take the lead to start needed centers, working in conjunction with each other where we could. Care Net's first focus was on Detroit, Michigan. Heartbeat decided to focus on Miami, Florida.

Miami had thirty-seven abortion clinics and not one pregnancy help medical clinic, that is, a help center with ultrasound services under the direction of a physician medical director. Rev. John Ensor from Boston, who had since joined the Heartbeat International Board, felt called to resign from the board and lead the Heartbeat project in Miami. John visited the area several times to understand the situation more fully, setting up an office each time, with his laptop, in Panera Bread. Finally, John and his wife Kristen decided that the only way to be successful in "waking up" the churches would be for them to move to Miami and become a part of the community for at least two years, which they did. The result is Heartbeat of Miami, two pregnancy help medical clinics (with ultrasound) that serve Hialeah (a Latino area with seven abortion clinics) and North Dade (an African American community with six abortion clinics), led by an outstanding leader who gave up a lucrative business position to answer the call to serve, Martha Avila.

John discovered that the Catholic Church in the Miami area, well aware of the abortion problem, had been struggling to keep several help centers functioning for years. They provided primarily material aid and referrals for community help. The Evangelical churches were largely unaware. So, John spoke at one or more churches in Miami every weekend, and sometimes during the week, calling attention to the problem and challenging Christians to answer the call. Innocent blood was being shed. Christians must act, as neighbors helping neighbors, getting involved like the Good Samaritan.

At one of the first churches, a woman named Jeannie Pernia came up to John after the service and said, "I was part of the problem—my mother and I ran one of the abortion clinics in Miami for several years—now I want to be part of the solution." Jeannie is now the director of the Hialeah pregnancy help clinic. When the site for the clinic was chosen, Jeannie told John that the abortion clinic she operated had been directly next door! How God heals and restores!

In an encouraging example of Christian unity, both Catholic and Evangelical churches actively support Heartbeat of Miami. I was greatly moved when I had the honor of participating at the grand opening of Heartbeat of Miami's first clinic, in Hialeah, in July 2007. The Archbishop of Miami, the Vicar of the Catholic Archdiocese, and seven Evangelical pastors attended the prayer service, a wonderful example of the Christian unity and "contending together" that Heartbeat hopes to model (see chapter 8).

The strategically located clinics of Heartbeat of Miami see about fifteen abortion-minded or abortion-vulnerable women every day. Most of whom decide to continue their pregnancies. The ultrasound images are not enough in and of themselves to help a woman choose life when she is faced with poverty, abandonment, coercion, fear, and other pressures. The women who come to Heartbeat of Miami (and other pregnancy help clinics around the world) are also enveloped in love and support, and provided with follow-up, hope, prayer, and practical help—the "weapons" of the army of foot soldiers armed with love.

The key to the development of pregnancy help centers and clinics in areas of greatest need, and perhaps the key to ultimate victory in the pro-life cause here in the

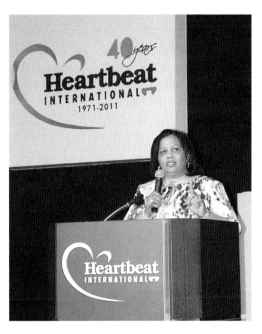

▲ *Sylvia Johnson receives one of Heartbeat's inaugural Legacy Awards at the Fortieth Anniversary Heartbeat International Conference in 2011 for her heroic work in urban pregnancy help centers. She is executive director of Downtown Pregnancy Help Center in Houston, Texas, only three miles from the largest abortion clinic in the United States, operated by Planned Parenthood.*

United States, is the leadership of the African American and Latino community. At Heartbeat, we call this group of leaders the "third wave" (to join the Catholic Christians of the "first wave" and the Evangelical Christians of the "second wave"). In the last five years, we have intentionally developed our "third wave" leadership within Heartbeat. For example, about 30 percent of all presentations at the Heartbeat International conferences are now given by Latino and African American leaders within our movement.

While others can provide a catalyst, resources, and vital support, pregnancy help centers in Latino and African American communities must be led by and "owned" by members of those communities. Dr. Alveda King, a member of the Heartbeat International Board who has dedicated her life to awakening the African American community to the harsh reality of abortion, illustrates the need for this when she says, "You can't go into someone's house, tell him he has a problem and that you know how to solve it better than he does."

One of the outstanding urban pregnancy help leaders in our movement today is Sylvia Johnson of Houston, Texas. Heartbeat honored Sylvia with a Legacy Award at our Fortieth Anniversary Conference for her courage and professionalism in leading pregnancy help ministry in a major, urban, abortion "hot zone." Sylvia is a founder of LEARN, one of the first African American, pro-life Christian organizations in the country. She directed a pregnancy help center in Orlando and then, in 2001, was moved to start the first urban center in what Houston's mayor described as the "forgotten part of the city." She is now the executive director of Houston Pregnancy Help Center with two locations, one only three miles from the largest abortion facility in the United States, the 78,000-square-foot Planned Parenthood abortion clinic, complete with a surgical wing for later term abortions. Sylvia Johnson is a courageous foot soldier, and she has raised up hundreds of others to fight alongside her, loving thousands of women into choices for LIFE.

There are many other long-serving men and women within Heartbeat International who lead other foot soldiers in their own cities (see appendix II). It is one of Heartbeat's major goals to raise up additional warriors, especially in the third wave of African American and Latino leaders within our movement, who can and will take back our major cities for life, and provide hope and positive alternatives for those most vulnerable to abortion.

Modeling Unity

Sometimes people say, "Why don't all you pro-life groups just get together?" The variety of groups in the pro-life movement evidently seems very confusing to the pro-life public. Well, there are probably lots of answers to that question, and I have wondered sometimes about all this myself, having been inside the pro-life movement since that fateful day, January 22, 1973. So, as an "insider" in the pro-life movement, here are my thoughts.

First, there are many different strategies that have proven effective within the overall pro-life mission in the United States. I will take a "stab" at articulating that overall mission: to promote the value of the sanctity of every human life in our culture, and especially, since abortion is the most horrendous and widespread attack on innocent human life, to reduce the number of abortions and eventually eliminate abortion as a legal option here and around the world. Another all-inclusive way of stating the overall mission has come into widespread use. It was first used by John Paul II in his 1994 encyclical, The Gospel of Life, or *Evangelium Vitae*: to turn from a culture of death and create a Culture of Life.

Strategies related to the broad anti-abortion mission have sometimes been divided into two types. The first type is strategies that attack the supply side, the availability of abortion: pass laws restricting and eventually outlawing all abortion, enforce strict licensing on abortion clinics, uncover abuses and get abortionists out of business, boycott businesses that give money to pro-abortion organizations, take our tax dollars away from Planned Parenthood, which owns the largest chain of abortion clinics in the United States and funds abortion around the world, and more.

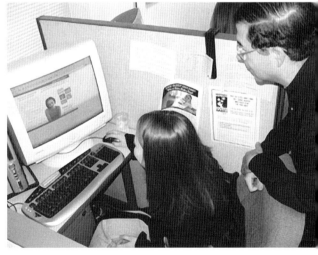

▲ *Father Frank Pavone, a major proponent of Option Line, visits the call center and observes a staff person at work, searching by zip code, to find the closest pregnancy help center for someone who has called the toll-free phone number. Option Line, co-founded by Heartbeat in 2003, has increased unity in the pregnancy help movement.*

The second type is strategies that reduce the demand side: pass laws that require waiting periods and informed consent so women have information to make better choices, inform women of their legal right NOT to be forced into an abortion, inform the general public about what abortion is and about its effects on babies, women, the entire family, and culture, provide a myriad of incentives so that women choose to have their babies, provide help and support so that woman do not feel that abortion is their only alternative, make ultrasound available to diagnose pregnancy early on with the result that both mothers and fathers can bond with their babies while they are in the womb, and more. According to this thinking, the pregnancy help movement would be one of the strategies attacking the demand side of abortion.

A third strategy is prayer and fasting. The Bible tells us, "If my people, who are called by my name, will humble themselves and pray and seek my face and turn from their wicked ways, then will I hear from heaven and will forgive their sin and will heal their land" (2 Chron. 7:14, NIV).

Pro-life organizations have emerged to take up each one of the above strategies. No country in the world except the United States, with its entrepreneurialism and "can do" attitude, with its freedom of speech, system of local, state, and federal laws, judicial system, tradition of philanthropy, predominant Judeo-Christian culture (for the time being), and its myriad of Christian churches, could ever generate the large number of pro-life organizations and individuals who feel called into this movement. Pro-life people in other countries are astounded at the pro-life activity and diversity in the United States. This is a good thing!

This diversity and overlapping of efforts that appear to some to be counterproductive may, in fact, be the kind of energy and dynamism that is the mark of workings of the Holy Spirit! The pro-life movement cannot be stamped out—there are simply too many of us, moving in too many directions. Eliminate some, but others will immediately take their place. One will fall, but others will jump in to raise the flag and march on. The disunity that many perceive in the movement is sometimes, no doubt, the work of the devil, but it may also be the protection of God.

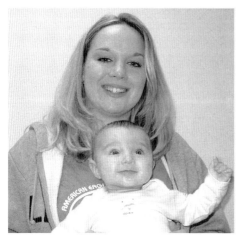

◀ *Alicia, who saw the Option Line phone number advertised on television one night when she was sleepless and worried about being pregnant, is one of the close to 1.4 million contacts who have reached Option Line since its founding. Connected to Pregnancy Decision Health Centers in Columbus, Ohio, she came into that pregnancy help medical clinic the next morning where she met with Peggy Hartshorn, who was volunteering that day. Alicia made a decision for life and is pictured with her baby Alexis. Alicia saved her baby's life, but she says Alexis saved her life too—she turned her life around, finished college, has a good job, and is a happy mother.*

Moreover, there is much more coordination and collaboration that takes place among the many organizations in our movement than most people realize. This includes regularly scheduled meetings of national leaders and several attempts through the years to develop overarching strategic plans.

Another logical division of the pro-life forces is this: there is the political, legislative, and educational arm of the movement, and it works primarily with the general public, legislators, and the courts. Then there is the service arm—the arm that provides help to those vulnerable to abortion and those who have suffered already from abortion; this arm works primarily with people one-on-one. These can also be thought of as the Justice and the Compassion arms of the movement.

Heartbeat International represents the Compassion arm of the movement, with nearly 1,200 pregnancy help centers and medical clinics, maternity homes, nonprofit adoption agencies, and abortion recovery programs in fifty countries. We estimate that we have about 25,000 volunteers, foot soldiers armed with love, working at any one time currently within our Heartbeat army.

"Anti-abortion" does not fully describe our compassion mission. "Pro-Life," in the fullest sense of the word, does describe us: we not only protect and defend the physical life of the unborn, but also the life and health (physical, emotional, psychological, and spiritual) of the mother and family, and we do this in a Christ-centered way. God is love, and love is our way, our "weapon" in this battle. To provide compassion means to "feel with" another, to enter into their suffering, and to minister to them through and with the love of Christ.

Heartbeat International has several national and international allies in the Compassion arm of the pro-life movement, each with a different approach, emphasis, or constituency. We are intentional about working in unity with them. As you can imagine, the devil would like nothing better than to spread discord among these groups since we are all saving women and babies from abortion daily. So Heartbeat has taken the lead to create as much collegiality, collaboration, and unity as possible throughout our forty-year history.

Lore Maier was fond of saying, "There can never be too many pregnancy help centers. There can never be any competition among us." She and our other founders were the first people to intentionally spread the vision of forming a variety of independent pregnancy help centers across the United States and around the world, traveling extensively at their own expense, offering services and affiliation with AAI, but realizing that not all centers would find a "home" in AAI. AAI materials and training were available to any center, regardless of affiliation. When Christian Action Council decided to "plant" a specific type of pregnancy center, each with an Evangelical statement of faith, Lore and Dr. John invited their executive director, Curtis Young, onto the AAI Board to learn whatever he could to help in the mission of Christian Action Council (now Care Net). For many years, AAI welcomed Birthright centers (that follow a franchise model with a strict charter of their own) to be part of AAI, and many did until the mid-1980s when Birthright directed their centers to affiliate and collaborate only with the Birthright "parent" organization, and this became part of the requirement of the Birthright charter.

So, when I became president in 1993, the value of unity was an essential part of Heartbeat's identity. We never were and never should be in competition with any other part of the compassion arm of the pro-life movement. Disunity among Christians is something that deeply pains our Lord. He emphasized His desire that we remain as one on the night before He suffered and died for our sins (disunity among Christian brothers and sisters being among those sins): "I pray also for those who will believe in me through their word, that all may be one as you, Father, are in me, and I in you; I pray that they may be one in us, that the world may believe that you sent me" (John 17:20–21, NAB). Unity is so important because, as Jesus tells us, this unity is necessary in order for the world to believe in Him.

Three things in Heartbeat International history since 1993 make me especially thankful about Heartbeat's role in guarding and modeling unity in our movement: "Our Commitment of Care" that became the "Our Commitment of Care and Competence"; the formation of the Leadership Alliance of Pregnancy Care Organizations; and Option Line, a joint venture between Heartbeat and Care Net for nearly ten years.

Our Commitment of Care and Competence

In 2001, Heartbeat gathered together with several other organizations in the compassion arm of our movement to discuss an ethical code of practice for pregnancy help centers, especially as it related to how we care for the women and others that the Lord sends to us. We started with the six affiliation principles of Heartbeat International (see chapter 5) and worked from there to develop a list of principles that we called "Our Commitment of Care."

This was then signed onto by all the existing membership groups of centers except Birthright (that agreed with the standards but declined to sign on, pointing to the requirement in their charter mentioned above). The signatory groups agreed to promulgate "Our Commitment of Care" among the centers that were part of their networks and make them a standard for affiliation.

As our relationships with these organizations continued to grow, it became clear that we agreed not only on guidelines that related to how we cared for the client but also on common operational guidelines that related to governance, fundraising, and medical services (pertinent laws and medical standards of care). In 2009, Heartbeat International proposed that additional standards be added to "Our Commitment of Care," and we arranged for input from all the original signatories and other pertinent partners. The updated document, called "Our Commitment of Care and Competence," has been signed onto by all the national organizations that provide affiliation, training, or resources for pregnancy help centers and clinics (with the continuing exception of Birthright) (see appendix VI).

When there are wild accusations made by those who want to close us down (see chapter 11) that pregnancy help ministries are, by their very nature, coercive, misleading, or even harmful to women, we can point to "Our Commitment of Care and Competence," our statement of ethical principles, that is posted in client care offices throughout the country.

Leadership Alliance of Pregnancy Care Organizations

Heartbeat International has also been a crucial partner in the development of an alliance that unites the national organizations that are part of the compassion arm of the pro-life movement. I was one of the founding members, and the alliance is still strong today.

The alliance grew out of a series of conflict resolution meetings among three national organizations. Julie Parton, then head of the pregnancy help ministry of Focus on the Family, and Anne Pierson, founder of Loving and Caring, brought the organizations together for a peacemaking effort in Lancaster, Pennsylvania. With much hard work, pain, and prayer, the conflict eventually was resolved. Out of that opportunity to pray together and develop personal relationships grew a natural desire to work more in harmony with each other and try to avoid disunity and conflict in the future.

On January 8, 2000, again in Lancaster, Pennsylvania, thirteen organizations that work in the compassion arm of the movement met together with a prayer leader and intercessor. We decided to meet again and to develop a more formal group that is now called the Leadership Alliance of Pregnancy Care Organizations. Our mission is this: "We exist to glorify God by joining in prayer and worship, discerning God's will, promoting and guarding unity, discussing, and developing collaborative relationships among leaders of national pregnancy care ministries."

Nothing like our Leadership Alliance exists in any other part of the pro-life movement. We get together annually for a full two days of relationship building, being hosted by a different member organization of our group each time. On the first day, we devote ourselves entirely to prayer. The form that this day takes depends on the hosting organization, and we have sometimes devoted an entire day to one purpose, such as repentance, or we have spent time in several types of prayer, such as adoration, contrition, thanksgiving, and supplication. The second day of our meeting is devoted to sharing information or discussing issues that affect the compassion arm of the movement, or participating in a leadership training opportunity planned by one of the member organizations.

A member cannot attend day two unless he or she has attended day one, the prayer day. We eat together, sometimes gather in smaller groups for networking or games, and generally get to know each other and enjoy one another's company. We commit to challenge each other when there is an issue that has threatened unity (not just brush dirt under the carpet), to walk humbly before God, and to not be satisfied with artificial politeness that covers an underlying breach. We have not always perfectly lived up to those goals, but we try.

I believe that the Lord has truly blessed the pregnancy help movement through the years in part because of our desire to be united, as He would have us be. Whenever I am present when other pro-life groups gather and disunity is evident, I share our experience with the Leadership Alliance, and challenge other pro-life organizations to begin praying together. I believe that our emphasis on a full day of prayer, each time we meet, is the key to working together cooperatively and collaboratively, despite our differences in mission, strategy, and methods. An added benefit is that the close relationships we have built have led to some strategic joint efforts, the most powerful being Option Line.

Option Line

A great example of unity in the pro-life movement, lasting nearly ten years with outstanding results, is Option Line, started as a joint venture managed and funded by Heartbeat International and Care Net. Option Line is promoted by other pro-life organizations and by pro-life advertisers (who add the Option Line number to their ads), and is found on billboards, in church bulletins, and in many other places. Option Line saves lives.

The Option Line call center started in January of 2003. Since then, Heartbeat and Care Net have marketed a toll-free phone number that is answered 24/7 by a specially hired and trained team of Christian women consultants, able to handle phone calls and other contacts in English and Spanish. We also market a cutting-edge website that attracts not only phone calls from those in need, but also contacts from email, instant messaging, and live chat. From January 2003 through the first quarter of 2011, Option Line has handled nearly 1.4 million contacts! Our goal is to reach as many people as possible who are vulnerable to abortion, let them know about their alternatives, and connect them to their local pregnancy help center, medical clinic, or post-abortion recovery program.

Option Line connects those in need, especially those vulnerable to abortion, to about 85 percent of all the pregnancy help centers in the United States and Canada. International contacts are referred to Heartbeat's international network through our *Worldwide Directory* online. With a MapQuest-type system, visitors to the website can also locate the closest center to them by typing in their zip code. In a web-based program that is growing rapidly, called Plus Link, Option Line is even able to make appointments for clients in many centers and clinics if their offices are closed at the time.

Why is this important? The Holy Spirit has raised up thousands of pregnancy help centers in our nation, but there was nothing linking this network together in an effective, professional way, and making it easy to access the services of our centers and clinics, until Option Line. And the battle is on between what abortion clinics offer and what our centers and clinics offer! It calls to mind Deuteronomy 30:19 (NIV): "I have set before you life and death, blessings and curses. Now choose life, so that you and your children may live."

We know that, for example, if a woman is considering abortion or is vulnerable to abortion (facing pressure from parents, boyfriend, financial concerns, and other issues) and she comes into a pregnancy help medical clinic for a medical diagnosis of pregnancy through ultrasound, there is an 80 percent chance (or higher) that she will choose life for her baby. The bonding begins to take place between mother and child, and her maternal instinct helps the mother protect her baby and not be overcome with fears and other pressures. The same often holds true for a father who, when he sees the image of his child on the ultrasound screen, often begins to fight to protect his child. But, if the mother gets to an abortion clinic first, we suspect that 80 percent of the time (some women do have the courage to walk out of an abortion clinic) she will go through with the abortion, the baby will be killed, and chances are that the mother and family will be left with physical, emotional, and/or spiritual scars. Who will get to the woman first?

Option Line now handles about 240,000 contacts each year (phone calls, emails, chats, instant messages). This is 20,000 per month, about 600 per day. Our goal is to increase that number dramatically as we learn more about marketing Option Line in a variety of ways and engaging the younger generation that spends so many hours per day on their cell phones and on the web. We are committed to continually "reinvent" Option Line so that it only increases its effectiveness in saving lives, in partnership with our pregnancy center network.

We sometimes hear back from the women we have helped through Option Line, often through email or instant messaging. Here is a "thank you" from March 15, 2010:

> *10:34 pm: are u there? Baby preston is Finally here . . . I love him so much . . . He is my everything!*
>
> *Answers at OL 1 10:35 pm: yes, I'm here. How can I help you today*
>
> *10:35 pm: I gave birth on the 11th with a beautiful baby boy . . . I just wanted to thank you for all the help you had to offer*
>
> *Answers at OL1 10:41 pm: we are glad we were here to help*

For me, the Option Line mission is especially personal. In 1980, my husband and I had the hotline for our Columbus pregnancy help center installed in our bedroom until the office was officially opened on January 22, 1981. We had to have a phone installed someplace by a certain date in order to get the number in the phone book. Unbeknownst to us, once installed, the number was accessible by operators when anyone called "Information" and asked about abortion! For several months, Mike and I learned "on the job" and answered many a desperate caller considering abortion. My resolve became firm that every call from a woman (or other person) vulnerable to abortion, at any hour of day or night, must be answered by a trained person who can provide help. If a woman has the courage to call, we must be there to answer. Now, that is exactly what happens nationwide and in Canada through Option Line.

I don't get to meet many of the mothers and babies who are saved through Option Line, but I have met and cared for one, and she is very dear to me. A few years ago, I was still working as a client care volunteer at our Heartbeat affiliate in Columbus. When I arrived for my scheduled volunteer time, my first appointment was with Alicia. Imagine my excitement when she indicated that she had called Option Line the night before, about 2:00 a.m., after seeing an Option Line ad on her TV! She was up late, worrying, and had just gotten home from an all-night drug store where she purchased two pregnancy tests. She could not believe the results (positive!), so when she saw the Option Line ad, she decided to call the number.

Option Line transferred her to our local center, and there she was in our office the next day! She knew that her own father and the father of the child would pressure her toward abortion, she would probably lose her job, and she might be thrown out of her home. She was willing to have an ultrasound to determine if she had a viable uterine pregnancy. Alicia is now the happy mother of Alexis. Her parents have become very supportive. She lives independently, is finishing college, is employed, and is a great mother. Thanks be to God for our local Heartbeat affiliates (in this case, Pregnancy Decision Health Centers), for Option Line, and for all the foot soldiers armed with love, all over the world, ready to minister to women like Alicia.

Defending Against Attack

Who would be against the work of pregnancy help centers that provide alternatives and support so that no woman ever feels that abortion is her only alternative? Who would attack those armed only with love? Even most pro-abortion leaders contend that no woman really wants to have an abortion, that those who do choose abortion have concluded that they have no other options. Former President Bill Clinton went so far as to declare that abortion should be "safe, legal, and rare."

Our founders thought that even people who declared themselves "pro-choice" (once that term was coined) would want to support pregnancy help centers. After all, these are the places where a variety of choices can be considered, as real alternatives to abortion, and these options can be worked through with caring, loving, and nonjudgmental help and support—single parenting, marriage, adoption, foster care, community resources to help with finances, housing, prenatal care, and more. Doesn't everyone agree that this is a good thing?

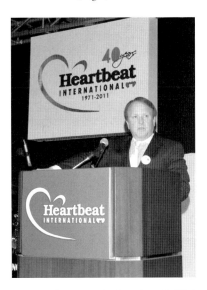

▲ Tom Glessner, J.D., founder of NIFLA and former Heartbeat International Board member, receives one of Heartbeat's inaugural Legacy Awards at the Fortieth Anniversary Heartbeat International Conference in 2011 for his pioneering work in developing the pregnancy help medical clinic with ultrasound services. Ultrasound has helped save thousands of lives yearly, and the professionalism brought by the medical model has helped protect our centers from attack.

Unfortunately, that has not been the case. Our opposition, headed by Planned Parenthood and NARAL Pro-Choice America, has orchestrated a number of attacks against pregnancy help centers and pregnancy help medical clinics, beginning in the early 1980s and continuing through today. They have attempted to smear us in the media, enact restrictive laws at the local, state, and federal level, and file harassing lawsuits against us.

Their motives are partly financial, since every mother who chooses life for her baby will not be one who pays for an abortion. They are partly political, since many of the legislators and attorneys general who have led attacks on centers have made promises to pro-choice organizations that help elect them. And their motives are partly personal. No doubt, many of those who lead the fight against our centers have been involved in abortions for themselves or others, and have an emotional stake in legitimizing that choice. We can't know all their motives for sure, but one thing that we do know is that their public motive— to "protect" women from being hurt by our centers and clinics—is a false one. No woman has been hurt or injured in one of our pregnancy centers or clinics. Compare this to documented cases of many women killed in "safe, legal" abortions in the United States.

As God would have it, these attacks that were meant for evil have actually strengthened our pregnancy help centers and our movement. The first example of that are the attacks in the 1980s that focused on the charge of "misleading advertising" and "fake clinics." In the early 1980s, Planned Parenthood of New York City hired Amy Sutnick for the specific purpose of finding a way to discredit pregnancy centers. Her efforts included charges of "deceptive advertising," alleged illegal practice of medicine, and the fact that our centers are religiously based, so not to be trusted.

Sending fake clients into our centers with hidden tape recorders and cameras in the 1980s was common. Both Ohio's attorney general (who later became the lieutenant governor) and the New York attorney general tried to restrict the advertising of our centers in the Yellow Pages. New York was successful, resulting in restrictions in that city and intimidation in many other places. Meanwhile, in California, Gloria Allred took action against the Right to Life League centers in the Los Angeles area, and a court in Los Angeles County ruled that doing pregnancy tests in centers was tantamount to "practicing medicine without a license."

Eventually, in the early 1990s, Mike Wallace did a hit piece on our centers on *Prime Time Live*, painting them as unprofessional, deceptive, anti-woman, and "fake clinics." In 1992, Oregon Congressman Ron Widen launched an investigation of pregnancy resource centers in the United States Congress, and he conducted a congressional hearing to document charges against our centers. He would not allow one person from pregnancy help centers to testify!

I was just becoming president of Heartbeat International about this time, and I was looking for legal help and advice, both for Heartbeat and our centers. How could we protect ourselves from more attack? How could we increase our professionalism and improve training of our staff and volunteers? How could we avoid charges that we had false advertising, or that we harassed clients? How could we avoid the charge of practicing medicine without a license?

Carol Aronis, the Cincinnati pregnancy center director whom God had used to encourage me to answer His call and become the leader of Heartbeat, was also the instrument He used to introduce me to Tom Glessner, J.D., who had been in the movement for many years. Tom was going to be in Cincinnati, and Carol encouraged us to meet and have lunch, which we did.

I learned that Tom and his wife Laura had started a center in Seattle, where Tom, an attorney in private practice, had been chairman of the board, and his wife had been the director of the center. They had personally experienced attacks on their center in the 1980s. They moved to the

Washington, D.C., area, and Tom had become the president of Christian Action Council, but Congressman Ron Widen had refused to let him testify at the congressional hearings.

We were all frustrated and afraid for the future of our centers. The attacks were front and center in Tom's mind and heart, so he had decided to devote himself entirely to providing legal help to our movement through a new organization he was founding. It was to be called NIFLA, National Institute of Family and Life Advocates.

Tom and I decided to partner our two organizations, NIFLA and Heartbeat International. We were both forming boards at that time, so we agreed to serve on each other's boards. We would encourage joint affiliation so centers would have the benefits of both Heartbeat's expertise and NIFLA's expertise. We partnered for about six years, as both organizations grew rapidly. Tom came to Heartbeat International conferences and taught our centers good legal practices and how to protect themselves to the greatest extent possible. With insurance expert and pro-life advocate Rick Renzi, Tom pioneered the first insurance program that was opened to all centers and published the first legal manual. Tom still teaches at Heartbeat conferences, and we work closely with him on many issues and projects, including recurring attacks on centers.

But the contribution that Tom has made to our movement, for which we recently honored him with our Legacy Award, is that he pioneered the use of ultrasound, so familiar now, in our pregnancy help medical clinics. It is hard to imagine that this concept was revolutionary in 1994. Tom and I were on each other's boards when Tom first proposed that our centers could become actual "medical clinics," under a physician medical director (volunteer), and provide "limited ultrasound," that is, an ultrasound exam for a limited purpose: to diagnose a viable uterine pregnancy (that is, a pregnancy that appears to be proceeding normally, one that is not ectopic or in the process of a natural miscarriage).

Knowing if she has a viable uterine pregnancy is a crucial piece of information if a woman is considering an abortion. If the pregnancy is not viable, there is no "need" for an abortion, and there were even documented cases of abortion clinics performing abortions on women who were not pregnant at all. (Tests of the "contents of the uterus" at labs confirmed that there was no embryo in the uterus at the time of the abortion.) Moreover, medical journal articles had documented that ultrasound examinations resulted in early bonding between mother and child. Clear recognition that the embryo or fetus was indeed real was also a vital piece of information for a person making a potential abortion decision.

Tom studied all the guidelines for use of ultrasound from the FDA, professional associations of ob-gyns, ultrasonographers, nurses, and others. He studied laws and medical standards of care. He finally published a medical "conversion" manual, which I also helped edit. I believed in Tom, NIFLA, and the model he proposed, and the pregnancy center that my husband and I helped found in Columbus, Ohio, was one of the first five centers in the country (in the mid-1990s) to purchase and use the ultrasound to help save and change lives. That center changed its name

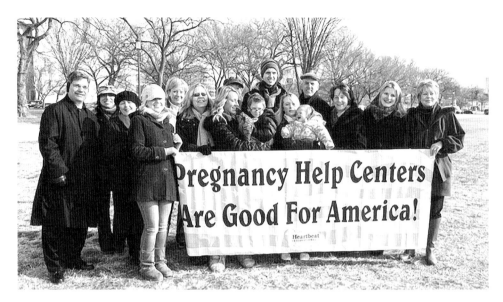

▲ *Heartbeat's "Babies Go to Congress" program is a pro-active way to make friends in Congress for our pregnancy help centers and help defend them from attack. In January each year, the "Babies Go to Congress" participants also attend the March for Life. Pictured here, with our March for Life banner, are some of the participants from 2011. L to R: Jor-El Godsey, Molly Hoepfner, Leslie Malek, Dawn Lunsford, Susan Dammann, Debbie Schirtzinger, Sasha Nelson, Charlie Nelson, Garrett Roney, Ahna Roney, Emma Roney, Rev. John Ensor, Peggy Hartshorn, Marilou Van Dongen, Peggy Benicke.*

from Pregnancy Distress Centers to Pregnancy Decision Health Centers. Other centers using ultrasound, also under the direction of a (volunteer) physician as medical director, began to use the term "medical" and "clinic" in their names.

Heartbeat eventually sponsored an annual Medical Clinic Symposium for a number of years to gather together our affiliates that were providing ultrasound services. In keeping with Heartbeat values, we asked our entrepreneurial affiliates to share how they were expanding the medical vision, and we brought other experts to stretch our thinking and help develop expanded models of medical services. These kinds of gatherings helped encourage some of our affiliates to add even more services such as STD testing and treatment, limited prenatal care, napro-technology (to teach patients about their reproductive health and treat certain medical conditions of the reproductive system), and even perinatal hospice (support for families who chose life, not abortion, after their baby was diagnosed with a condition that would likely result in death in the womb or soon after birth).

Heartbeat also researched and sponsored training for centers on how to bill for Medicaid services, if their volume of services warranted. The wide variety of medical services provided within pregnancy help medical clinics today, and the potential of these clinics in the future, is partly a result of Heartbeat's leadership and the pioneering and entrepreneurial spirit of our independent affiliates. We are willing to take risks, when guided by the Holy Spirit, to save lives in a life-changing way, and advance a Culture of Life.

So, ironically, the opposition charged us with being "fake clinics" (fake abortion clinics). But we responded with becoming actual clinics, medical clinics that provide a medical diagnosis of pregnancy through the use of a limited ultrasound exam, and more! This has made pregnancy help centers and clinics less vulnerable to attack and stronger than ever.

Attacks have continued, of course, even though many centers are now medical clinics operating under the license of a private physician, or licensed by their state (where that is required, especially in Massachusetts and California). In the 2000s, NARAL, the major lobbying partner of Planned Parenthood, published a guide on how to close down your local pregnancy center, and five similar guides were published by various NARAL state coalitions. The National Abortion Federation also released a "report" on the evils of pregnancy centers in 2006.

Moreover, in 2006, Congressman Henry Waxman (D-CA), then a member of the U.S. House of Representatives Committee on Government Reform, issued a rogue report entitled "False and Misleading Health Information Provided by Federally Funded Pregnancy Resource Centers." By the way, the federal funding referred to in the title was based on the fact that about one hundred pregnancy centers in the nation had received some federal funding for abstinence education programs in the schools in the faith-based funding programs promoted under the Bush administration; none of that funding was used in core center programs that the Waxman report cited as using "false and misleading health information."

Nothing will satisfy our opponents on the subject of "accurate medical information" it seems, unless we proclaim that abortion has absolutely no negative physical or psychological effects and that there is absolutely no statistical connection between abortion and breast cancer. However, these statements are not true, and we are committed to truth and accuracy. Women deserve it. All medical information used by Heartbeat in our training and materials is medically referenced and approved by Heartbeat's Medical Advisory Board, consisting of eight experts in the fields of obstetrics, gynecology, and radiology.

In 2002, New York's then attorney general, Eliot Spitzer (who fell from prominence as governor of New York because of a call girl scandal in 2008), orchestrated an attack all across New York, targeting twenty-four centers. In a major example of unity and cooperation, Heartbeat worked closely with our national partners and with local attorneys to unravel the strategy, and all charges were eventually dropped. This was miraculous but also exhausting.

After New York, it was clear that Heartbeat needed an attorney on staff to work with our centers on a regular basis, lead Heartbeat's center defense strategy, and work with our national partners when attacks occur. Peg Wolock was hired and worked tirelessly for about ten years, doing legal reviews for affiliates to be sure they were as strong as possible, and writing a legal manual, published jointly with Care Net. We now work with other partners such as Alliance Defense Fund, American Center for Law and Justice, Christian Legal Society, state Family Policy Councils, and Catholic Bishops' organizations, as needed and appropriate, when and where attacks occur.

In the past couple of years, there has been a flurry of attacks at the state and local level. Bills that would regulate and restrict our advertising (and potentially close down our centers) have been defeated in places such as Washington and Oregon, but the battles there have been hard-fought, and we do not expect our enemies to give up there. Bills have also been introduced, but never advanced, in Maryland, Texas, Virginia, and West Virginia.

Our opponents have hit upon a successful strategy, however, by introducing restrictive bills in cities and counties asserting, with no actual evidence, that our centers are "deceptive" and pose a threat to women. They quickly passed legislation between 2010 and 2011 in Austin, Baltimore, Montgomery County (outside Washington, D.C.), and New York City. The New York bill, for example, requires that a New York City commissioner will promulgate rules for conspicuous signage for our centers, in English and Spanish, in a specific letter size and type, "warning" potential clients about what we do not do (for example, provide or refer for abortions or contraceptives). Penalties designated in the law, to be enforced by the New York City police department, involve fines, civil penalties, "sealing" the center, and even imprisonment!

We are fortunate that one of the laws has been found to be unconstitutional in the United States District Court for the District of Maryland, with the court finding that the Baltimore ordinance "violates the Freedom of Speech Clause of Article I of the Constitution of the United States of America and is unenforceable" (decision handed down on January 28, 2011). Common sense would tell us that this will slow down bills of this sort, but the New York City ordinance, even more restrictive than the Baltimore one, was passed *after* this court ruling was handed down. Mayor Bloomberg was heard to say by one of our center directors as he signed the New York City law, "It may be unconstitutional, but I'm signing it anyway." The harassment and smear campaign against us thus continues, motivated, it appears, not by any facts but by political pressure and paybacks.

By the grace of God, the attacks over the past thirty years have led to a high level of professionalism in all that we do in our centers and medical clinics. The attacks resulted directly in the vision for real clinics (with ultrasound) to counter the charge that we are "fake clinics." And I am sure that even more lives have been saved and changed as a direct result of our response to these attacks.

Heartbeat has always promoted the highest standards of training and education for our foot soldiers and the centers and clinics where they carry out their mission. Heartbeat's leadership in expanding "Our Commitment of Care and Competence" has already been discussed, as has our development of the first college-level, adult education, distance-learning training program for pregnancy consultants called ConCert, through Project REACH. We have gone "high tech" now with our distance-learning program, and we are transitioning all our core training to online, adult education modules, starting with *The LOVE Approach™*, which was completed this anniversary year.

Heartbeat has developed a suite of up-to-date training materials as companions to the 2011 edition of *The LOVE Approach:* a comprehensive board training manual called *GOVERN Well™* and a comprehensive director's manual called *DIRECT Well™*. In addition, we have a medical manual for centers that want to add medical services, a legal manual (published in 2011), and an up-to-date staffing manual, among other resources. We also provide a comprehensive, onsite center assessment, as well as

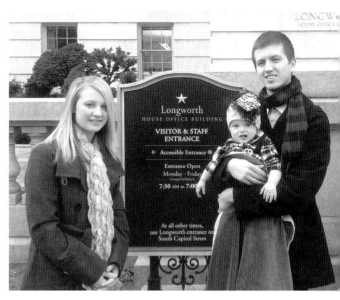

▲ *Garrett and Ahna Roney in front of the Longworth Building before they visit their congressional representative in January 2011. Their testimony of how the Pregnancy Care Center in Springfield, Missouri, helped them choose life and mentored them through a very difficult period is told in this chapter.*

strategic planning, peacemaking, and consultations personalized for special needs. Our unique Institute for Center Effectiveness and our New Director Oasis are specialized, intensive training opportunities for special groups of leaders within our movement.

A few years ago we launched a one-of-its kind certification program for our foot soldiers called the LAS certification, standing for Life Affirming Specialist™. After core training requirements, someone working in a center or clinic can obtain an LAS certification, given by a recognized provider that certifies courses for continuing education for professional counselors and social workers. By attending Heartbeat International conference workshops that meet certain standards, consultants in our centers obtain continuing education credits and keep up their certification as a Life Affirming Specialist. Recent conference tracks and workshops have also been approved for continuing education credits for nurses as well.

Attacks or no attacks, we believe it is important to do everything well, with the highest standards of excellence and integrity, and this is what we provide in all our training and support for our affiliates. Our main "weapon" in the battle continues to be truth in love. We are providing love and support, in ways that are above reproach, to women and families every day. And communities are stronger as a result.

This is the message, "Pregnancy centers are good for America," that Heartbeat takes to Washington, D.C., on a regular basis in our pro-active effort to make friends with influencers in our nation's capitol. At the national level we call our outreach "Babies Go to Congress®." We have also modeled the same approach at the Ohio legislature and called it "Babies Go to Columbus." It can be "Babies Go to Chicago" or any city that introduces legislation attacking our centers.

In our Babies Go to Congress program, Heartbeat makes an appointment with a member of Congress, or their Washington office staff, and we bring a mother and baby (or mother, father, and baby) who have been helped by a pregnancy center in their district. Also coming to the congressional office with the constituent mother and her baby is the director of the local center and a representative from Heartbeat International. Each mother tells her story of how the center has helped her, confirming that without the center's help this baby would likely have been aborted. Sometimes the babies, in strollers and carriers, chime in with their thanks too. The center director explains all the services provided at their center. Thus we all make friends for local pregnancy centers that provide a wide range of vital community services in their congressional districts, all at no cost to the taxpayers.

Over the past few years, Heartbeat has been able to visit more than 120 congressional offices and taken seventy moms and babies to Congress. We try to focus on pro-choice or noncommittal congressional representatives and senators, and we have almost invariably gotten a positive response. Legislators and their aides find it almost impossible to argue, once they have a mother and baby who are their own constituents in front of them, that the work of their local pregnancy center is anything other than a very good thing.

I have had the blessing of being with several mothers and babies when they visited Congress. In this anniversary year, I was with Cindi Boston, the executive director of our affiliate in Springfield, Missouri, who brought Garrett and Ahna and their baby to meet their congressional representative and tell their story. In July of 2009, Garrett and Ahna had both just turned seventeen and were seniors in high school. When they suspected that Ahna might be pregnant, according to Garrett, "We were terrified about what would happen and how we would be viewed and if we would ever be able to make it." Happily, they found the pregnancy center instead of an abortion clinic, but they were still confused and frightened. The center matched Garrett with a mentor, and this is what Garrett says about their experience in his written testimony prepared for his congressman:

> At the Pregnancy Care Center, I was able to talk to my mentor and get his advice. You see, I loved Ahna very much, and I had planned on one day marrying her. I eventually proposed. We continued coming to the center for relationship classes, fatherhood classes, healthy pregnancy classes, and to see our mentor. With the help of Pregnancy Care Center and their wonderful staff and volunteers. Ahna and I were able to get the help and support that we so greatly needed. Now we have a beautiful daughter named Emma Grace. I know that our lives may have gone in a different direction if not for the center. I'm an 18-year-old husband and father, and it's the greatest experience. I know there will be challenges ahead, but the center has given us the tools to build a healthy relationship so we can build a healthy family whatever comes our way.

Advancing Globally

Globally, the number of abortions is staggering, and so is the need for pregnancy help services. For comparison, there are approximately 1.2 million surgical and medical abortions (RU486, the "abortion pill") each year in the United States, with about 25 percent of all pregnancies ending in abortion. (That rate is much higher in some major cities and among African Americans, Latinos, and some immigrant groups.) A conservative estimate of the number of abortions around the world each year is between forty-five and fifty million. In Russia, for example, there are about four times the number of abortions as live births, and in Vietnam, nine out of ten pregnancies ends in abortion.

The good news is that the Holy Spirit is working mightily and raising up thousands of people worldwide who are aware of the problem and are answering the call to help. Our best estimate (and a conservative one) is that there are nearly 2,000 pregnancy help centers outside the United States. It is difficult to keep track of the specifics of where and how the Holy Spirit is working, but when it comes to pregnancy centers around the world, Heartbeat tries! For nearly all of our history, we have published a *Worldwide Directory* of pregnancy help, listing locations of centers, maternity homes, and similar resources by country and city.

Some people now access this valuable tool for referral and networking via our website, www.heartbeatinternational.org,

▲ *First page of the original AAI directory, published on mimeographed sheets in February of 1972. It contained about 130 centers in the United States, 11 in Canada, and 1 in New Zealand.*

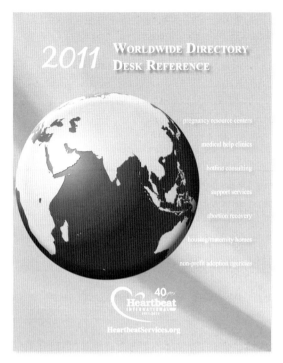

▲ Current Heartbeat International Worldwide Directory Desk Reference. The annual Worldwide Directory is also available on the Internet at www.heartbeatinternational.org. It contains 3,718 entries in the United States, and 1,747 in eighty-four other countries. The Worldwide Directory makes it possible for leaders to network with each other around the world, and it saves lives because women can be referred for service to the nearest pregnancy help center.

but others still use the paper version, the desk reference, and sometimes refer to it as a "phone book," like the pregnancy center director who sent us this recent email:

"Thank you for your International status and for that phone book [Heartbeat's 2010 Worldwide Directory*] that clutters my office!*

A few months ago, I received a call from a girl living in another state. She had found herself pregnant and was abortion minded…She knew me because I am friends with her family. What ensued was nothing short of a miracle. We had several conversations, and I was able to connect her with a pregnancy help clinic [in the Worldwide Directory*] in the city she lived—because of my Heartbeat family!…She has since chosen to adopt…*

Today, I received a phone call from a woman in another country that is not Christian friendly! A woman who had come into my clinic a while ago called because she needed a friend and had felt a connection with me as I was the one who had administered her pregnancy test. I was able to connect her with a place close to where she lives, once again, because of that phone book!

What a tool that phone book has proven to be—I am so grateful that I have this resource and am able to help others knowing that if they are in your phone book, they are legit and will help those in need—all around the world! What a blessing. Thank you so very much for the work you do as well as putting that resource together…I'm sure there are many stories of how God has used that phone book—well, here are 2 more to add!"

Forty years ago, our founders, especially Lore Maier, had a worldwide vision for the pregnancy help movement. As noted earlier in this history, almost immediately after adopting the name AAI at our founding in 1971, standing for Alternatives to Abortion Incorporated, Lore and Dr. John proposed changing our official name to Alternatives to Abortion International, and it was.

Lore, as the first executive director, wrote hundreds of letters to contacts around the world, sharing the vision. She and Dr. John traveled extensively, at their own expense, inviting others to start pregnancy help centers in their own nations and become part of the federation of AAI. These emerging leaders were invited to the annual AAI Academy and encouraged to participate fully as affiliates, and international leaders joined the AAI Board in the mid-1970s.

It became one of the goals of AAI to keep track of all the emerging service centers whether or not they became official affiliates. AAI published this *Worldwide Directory* of centers, national and international, each year starting in 1972. This first edition had about 130 entries in the United States, 11 in Canada, and 1 in New Zealand. Heartbeat International still keeps up this task. This year's *Worldwide Directory* contains 3,718 entries in the United States (including traditional pregnancy help centers and medical clinics, maternity support organizations, maternity homes and other residential programs, professional social service agencies, nonprofit adoption agencies, and abortion recovery programs) and 1,747 centers in eighty-four other countries (one-third of all the countries in the world).

Our Option Line (chapter 10) uses the online *Worldwide Directory* for referrals to centers outside the United States and Canada when requests for help are received through the Option Line website (www.optionline.org) from people who cannot be connected immediately to a U.S. or Canadian center.

Heartbeat International today, like we have done from the beginning of our history, responds with leadership training, resources, and individualized support whenever we are contacted by an emerging new center outside the United States. Today, most of these new centers are being started by indigenous groups, often called to action when Planned Parenthood or a United Nations–sponsored program comes into their region to liberalize abortion laws, ostensibly to take care of "hard cases" (such as rape or incest) or under the guise of "women's reproductive health care," much as they did in the United States in the late 1960s. (The real intention of most of these groups is, like it was in the United States, to radically change the sexual mores of the culture, taking away that culture's traditional moral and religious underpinning for marriage and the family.) Frequently, new international centers are envisioned, encouraged, and supported by missionaries from American churches who are assigned in that region of the world and see the need for centers where women can feel safe and be supported in their choice for life.

Just like in the United States, Heartbeat has found, however, that it is not enough to simply respond to those who initiate the contact and come to us for help in establishing pregnancy help centers. We must also go proactively to areas of greatest need, like we have here at home, to help the local church, the Body of Christ, understand the need and catch the vision. Then Heartbeat can provide help and support onsite to those who answer the call. We have had two successful

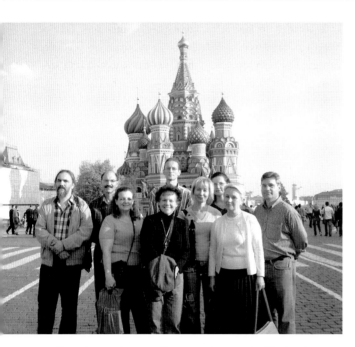

▲ *Heartbeat helps provide the training onsite for Russian pregnancy center leaders in 2007. Pictured in front of St. Basil's Cathedral in Red Square, Moscow, are Father Maxim Obukhov (Moscow, Russia), Bill Velker (Grand Rapids, MI), Carolyn Rice (Greenville, SC), Debbie Nieport (Dayton, OH), Alex Van Vuuren (Hilversum, Netherlands), Lena Batina (Kharkov, Ukraine), Jor-El Godsey (Heartbeat International, Columbus, Ohio), and other team members.*

experiences with conferences overseas, in partnership with LIFE International, one in Budapest and one in Ukraine. Each trained nearly one hundred people, primarily from Eastern Europe, who were working in existing ministries or hoping to start new ones.

Heartbeat International currently has about three hundred officially affiliated pregnancy help ministries in fifty countries outside of the United States, and we are working on specific strategies to either start or strengthen pregnancy help services on every continent (except Antarctica): North America (United States and Canada); South America; Europe (Western and Eastern); Asia; Africa; and Australia.

Heartbeat has been providing leadership training and mentoring for international pregnancy help leaders partly through our annual international training conference since 1995. Our international scholarship program provides support to cover part of the expenses of selected international leaders to get training at our conference and then visit and network with centers in the United States. International delegates raise support in their own countries for the other part of their expenses. About 175 individual leaders from forty-two countries have come to the United States to be trained by Heartbeat International over the past sixteen years, and some have made several trips here for additional training and mentoring.

We have special relationships in some parts of the world where there is a national or regional group of pregnancy help centers that, with help and support, can grow and develop more and stronger centers in partnership with Heartbeat International. In some cases, we have licensed our core training materials to organizations in those regions so they can be translated or modified to better suit the culture. These regions include Canada, Australia, Africa, Latin America, and the Philippines.

Lily Perez, along with her husband Rene, came to the Heartbeat International conference from the Philippines for the first time ten years ago. They were housing homeless pregnant girls in their own small home at that time. Their first girl had been brought to their home by a local taxi driver who almost ran over the girl when she was thrown by her husband "like a bowling ball in one of the alleys in Tondo" (says Lily). She was three months pregnant, and her husband wanted her to get rid of the baby. The driver knew about their pro-life work and asked Lily and Rene if they would help the girl. They did, and their ministry started from that day.

After being trained at the conference and afterwards for a week at the Heartbeat headquarters, Lily left with a passion to do even more in her homeland and her region of the world, along with the knowledge and tools to get started. Eventually, these formalized into the vision for the NGO (nonprofit organization) that she started, calling it Pregnancy Support Services of Asia. After years of praying, networking, and working to overcome one obstacle after another, Lily now has six centers affiliated with PSSA, and she has contacts who want to help start pregnancy help centers in several other regions of Asia.

Along with a Heartbeat consultant from Heartbeats of Licking County, Ohio, Rindy Brooks, I spent a memorable week in Manila in March 2006, training more than one hundred volunteers eager to work in pregnancy help centers all over the Philippines, and to help start centers regionally. This year, Lily met with people interested in beginning pregnancy help ministries in East Asia (Bangladesh, India, East Timor, Pakistan, and other countries).

The Philippines, Latin America, and parts of Africa are in the crosshairs of Planned Parenthood and other pro-abortion forces (who partner with the United Nations) since these places are among the last remaining predominantly Christian regions in the world. In these places, abortion has almost always been viewed as an abomination (as it is, of course). Sex education in the schools and free contraceptives are not yet the norm, as they are in many Western countries. Generally, children are still welcomed and valued. However, these values are changing, even as I write, and pro-life people are fighting desperately in these regions to preserve the legal protections still provided to human beings in the womb.

Having experienced the changes in American culture over the past forty years, I was amazed and awed when I visited Manila for the first time in 2001 at the invitation of Sister Pilar Versoza, head of Pro-Life Philippines, who was helping the mayor of Manila with "Pro-Life Week" in this major world city. There are only a few countries in the world, unfortunately, where a United States pro-life leader would be treated as an official dignitary! During that week, I had three or four speaking engagements every day, including community health clinics, schools, and universities. I helped dedicate a major pro-life sculpture in one of the city squares and a section of a large cemetery for the burial of babies found aborted (victims of illegal abortion). I was feted at City Hall and even given the key to the city of Manila by the mayor, and the Manila city band played "Stars and Stripes Forever" in my honor!

What an amazing experience for me to be in a country and city whose official stance was 100 percent pro-life. The mayor, a true believer in the value of every person, instituted many programs to help the poor maintain their dignity and earn a living. For example, a foundation for the blind that had trained its blind clients in head massage techniques was allowed to provide head massages (for a small donation) to people like me, who relaxed on a folding chair, during lunch hour, in a major Manila city square.

I saw things in the Philippines that touched me deeply, and showed me again how uniquely God's people respond to His call, depending on the specific needs of their country and their own culture. Even though abortion is still illegal in the Philippines, many desperate women are sold misoprostol (cytotec) on the streets (misoprostol-cytolec is an ulcer drug used off label to cause abortions), and they take this pill, which causes serious bleeding. I learned that a group of Filipino foot soldiers armed with love, called "Veronicas," visited hospitals to minister to women in the emergency rooms who are in the midst of abortions caused by misoprostol.

These women call themselves "Veronicas" after the woman who, in the tradition of the early church, wiped the face of Jesus as He carried His cross on the way to Calvary. Jesus left the image of His face on her cloth (*Vera iconica* means "true image"). They see Jesus' face in the suffering faces of the women who succumb to abortion out of desperation. People in the Philippines are responding with the message of love and hope in community pregnancy centers so that no woman will ever feel that abortion is her only alternative.

I and other members of the Heartbeat staff have made repeated trips to Africa where we are partnering with Africa Cares for Life, a vision of Gail Schreiner, who started a pregnancy help center in Durban, South Africa, about twenty years ago. It was the first pregnancy help center in Africa, as far as we know. Her example spread all over South Africa, and her vision is now to "fan the flames" and help centers grow and develop all over the continent. The level of personal sacrifice needed to do this work in other countries, including Africa, is moving and inspiring. Gail, for example, has worked without salary for more than twenty years, mostly out of her own home, supported primarily by her husband's generosity and a handful of other donors. Gail almost had an abortion about thirty years ago when her boyfriend took her from Africa to England for the "procedure." But she got off the abortionist's table and refused to kill her child, knowing that she would face the loss of her boyfriend, her job, and the support of her family. All of that did occur because of her choice for life. One woman, a Good Samaritan, however, took Gail into her own home and helped her through her pregnancy. That's how Gail knew there was a need for pregnancy centers. God finally moved her to start one, and she stepped out in faith and said "yes." Now there are nearly forty centers throughout South Africa and more starting in other African countries.

The forms that centers take in Africa are specific to their cultural needs. In Zambia, for example, Barbra Mwansa and her husband, Pastor Edward Mwansa, who were among the first international

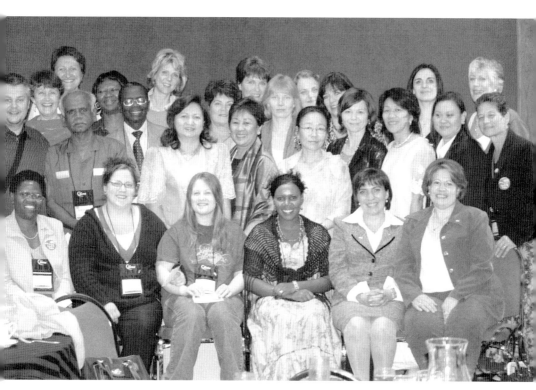

▲ Delegates from around the world, many thanks to scholarships provided through gifts from Heartbeat's generous partners (individuals, foundations, and our pregnancy center affiliates), attend the Heartbeat International Conference in 2008. Pictured, L to R: Bottom row: Julie Sibanda (Zimbabwe), Christin Newman (USA), Cami Kellenbarger (USA), Barbra Mwansa (Zambia), Lourdes Delgado (Mexico), Rossana Soto (Mexico). Middle row: Alexey Klimenko (Russia), Sam Jothimani (India), Purification Echiverri (Philippines), Lily Perez (Philippines), Lucita Tagle (Philippines), Vesna Nikolic (Serbia), Cherry Lynn Trinidad (Philippines), Julia Cardenal (El Salvador), Judy Vasquez (Belize). Top row: Paula Grimsley (USA), Lyuba Uryutova (Russia), Gladys Adochim (Ghana), Oliver Mulenga (Zambia), Shelly Crouch (Russia), Kathy Michel (Canada), Claudia Walter (Nepal), Lene Duechlom Hansen (Denmark), Kaisa Aardevalja (Estonia), Gail Schreiner (South Africa), Vesna Radeka (Serbia), Jennifer Street (New Zealand).

delegates ever to come to be trained by Heartbeat in the United States, have developed, over the years, a ministry that encompasses a traditional pregnancy help clinic with pregnancy testing and ultrasound services, plus an abstinence education program in the schools and a post-abortion program. But the ministry also has a maternity home (built with cement blocks made onsite by Barbra and Edward and their many volunteers, and added onto when they had the resources to make more blocks); an orphanage, where some of the children are HIV positive but, because of excellent care, cannot be distinguished from the other children; a feeding program for children that also teaches natural family planning for the mothers; and a boys' ranch to teach life skills to street boys. The Mwansas' work is supported by a for-profit business in Kitwe, local community donors, and churches, and nonprofit organizations from the United States.

In Eastern Europe, where Communism all but destroyed the family, many centers have been developed in Romania, Russia, the Ukraine, Hungary, Poland, and elsewhere. It was heartbreaking when one of our affiliates in Russia told me that the resource they needed most at their pregnancy center was videos or other materials they could use to show mothers how to touch and hold their babies. She told me that since abortion is so rampant (the average number of abortions per Russian woman is seven) and Communism put all mothers in the workforce and children in day-care centers, parents seem to have no innate parenting skills and need to be shown what, for most mothers and fathers, should come naturally.

Influencers in Russia are now trying to reverse the damage done, and they are uniting to try to reconstitute the Russian family and confront the "demographic winter" that is so evident there. This year, I had the blessing of giving a paper on "The Dignity of Women" at the Moscow Demographic Summit: The Family and the Future of Mankind, sponsored by the World Congress of Families, and endorsed by Russian government, industry, and Orthodox Church leaders. I also had the opportunity to network with one of the key leaders in pregnancy center development in Russia, Father Maxim Obukhov, with whom we plan to partner even more in the future.

In Asia, besides the Philippines, Heartbeat is working strategically in areas that must be kept confidential because of the persecution of Christians going on there. We have found that the dedicated Christians in "underground churches" are often totally ignorant of the facts of human development, and they have no concept of what abortion actually is—that abortion truly destroys a living, growing, human being in the earliest stages of development. They have no understanding of what the Bible teaches on the sanctity of every human life. When they know these truths, they are deeply repentant for their silence on abortion. Despite the risk to themselves, they are keenly motivated to become involved and to provide shelter and support for women who, often in ignorance, are being emotionally or physically coerced into abortions.

In the United States, with the vast amount of resources with which we have been blessed, we must make even greater efforts to share these resources with those overseas who are heroically stepping forward as foot soldiers armed with love. The challenges are daunting, but the Lord is great, and the opportunities are limitless for Christians to become involved with financial investment, prayers, and partnerships around the globe.

Digging to the Core

I personally was called into the pro-life movement early on (January 22, 1973) because I was alarmed and distraught to realize that "they are killing babies" and this is happening in my country, a Judeo-Christian country, one that is founded on the truth that "we are endowed by our Creator with certain inalienable rights," and the "right to life" is the first one (see introduction). My call, I believed, was to save as many lives as possible while working to return our country to our founding values as expressed in our Constitution and the law of the land. Over the last nearly forty years, the Lord has shown me that the core of my call and, I believe, the call of Heartbeat International, is even deeper. How I arrived at that realization and how Heartbeat International has moved deeper toward this core, in our vision, mission, and programming, is the story to be told in this chapter.

One of the aspects of the AAI Academy, the precursor to the Annual Heartbeat International Conference, that intrigued me when I first began attending them in the 1980s was the diversity of affiliates and the variety of programs they were providing. It was not just pregnancy testing and crisis intervention for women who were considering abortion, although this was the core service of centers (originally called E.P.S. centers, standing for Emergency Pregnancy Services). The foot soldiers in the field had begun to discuss and provide a wider range of help and support. For example, maternity homes were represented and presenting workshops on the importance of fatherhood and adoption into a two-parent family. Later in the 1980s, Anne and Jimmy Pierson were regulars at the AAI Academies with their message of the importance of family and the danger of fatherlessness.

Sister Paula, especially, emphasized the importance of our counseling sessions with women who had a negative pregnancy test (over 50 percent of all clients at that time). We were not called into action to help these clients choose life instead of abortion—they weren't pregnant. Instead, Sister Paula taught, we could help these women understand the danger to themselves as women of continuing in sexual activity outside of marriage. Remember, I mentioned earlier in this history that our early "negative test" counseling focused on the "psychology" of womanhood, not on sexually transmitted diseases (STDs) and the physical dangers of sexual activity with multiple partners because most STDs at that time could be cured with antibiotics, and HIV/AIDs was not even on the scientists' radar until 1981.

Soon, however, as the 1980s progressed and the epidemic of STDs began to reveal itself, and especially as HIV/AIDs became a scourge not only in the homosexual population but also spread into the heterosexual population, our negative test counseling became more and more focused on the dire physical risks of sexual activity outside of marriage. The deeper psychological and spiritual dimensions of that activity began to take less and less prominence in our conversations with clients. So, our training began to focus more and more on physical, medical risks for women.

In the 1980s, centers took their message out of the counseling centers and began teaching about abstinence until marriage in their community schools in an effort to help prevent the kinds of cases they were seeing in their pregnancy centers. At our annual gathering of affiliates, abstinence education programs began to be highlighted and taught. Because programs in public schools must be secular, most of the programs that centers developed were based on a medical model, teaching about STDs in order to deter sexual activity. Many added a relationship component and incorporated information and activities to teach young people about how to form a lasting relationship, noting that multiple sexual partners has the effect of numbing the ability to form long-term relationships, endangering the dream that young people still had, at that time, of someday finding the perfect person with whom they thought they would spend the rest of their life. Some programs were reluctant to discuss marriage per se (for fear of being ejected from the public schools), so they focused on a "lifetime monogamous relationship" in their teaching.

In fact, the abstinence education movement, so prominent in our country today, was birthed out of AAI pregnancy help centers in the 1980s. The center my husband and I helped found in Columbus was the first center in the country to receive a federal grant for abstinence education through a "model program" initiative started by pro-life appointees in the U.S. Department of Health and Human Services (HHS), as part of the Office of Family Planning during the Reagan administration in 1984. I knew a former Right to Life leader, Margery Mecklenburg, who was working in Washington for HHS, and I called to ask if any funding was available through the government. She told me about the experimental program. Our pregnancy center applied, went through a competitive grant review process, and received a three-year grant, beginning in 1984. Our opponents later challenged this program in the courts as a violation of the separation of church and state, and our pregnancy center was involved in depositions for the court case. It was eventually decided in our favor, and the concept was upheld that faith-based organizations can receive federal funding for programs, as long as those programs do not "proselytize."

This Supreme Court decision paved the way for the Bush-era expansion of the faith-based initiatives that made millions of dollars available for abstinence education in our schools. After that first grant in 1984, I served as an advisor for a number of years to the U.S. Department of Health and Human Services, in the Office of Family Planning, and was a grant reader on panels that rated proposals from all over the country for abstinence education grants. I am grateful to the Reagan administration for intentionally training me and many other pro-life leaders at that time in how the government awards grants and how we can become competitive in the process.

The HHS oversight process of grantees was a tremendous asset in helping our center grow in professionalism, especially in our accounting and administrative processes. Eventually, more than one hundred pregnancy help centers received federal funding (either directly from HHS or through block grants to their states) for abstinence education in their communities during the George W. Bush administration. A few have received grants through later Bush programs under "fatherhood initiatives" and "marriage initiatives" to promote and strengthen marriage in their communities.

When I became president of Heartbeat in 1993, I remember calling Leslee Unruh, the director of our affiliate in Sioux Falls, South Dakota, whom I met and worked with during the time that both of our pregnancy centers were receiving abstinence funding and developing excellent abstinence education programs. I suggested that perhaps she could help me identify, for purposes of our *Worldwide Directory*, all the centers that provided abstinence education, along with the new free standing abstinence education programs in the country. Leslee later shared with me

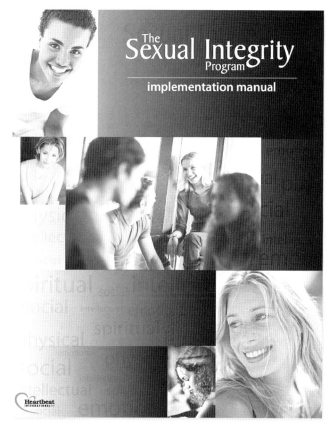

▲ Heartbeat's Sexual Integrity Program is unique in the pregnancy help movement. It provides training on how to introduce the concept of sexual integrity, or sexual wholeness, to our clients, and it includes a wide range of tools, including brochures, charts, books, video components, and workbooks on healing from sexual abuse, fertility appreciation, and the beauty of marriage. This program gets to the core of God's Plan for Our Sexuality, often an entirely new vision for those the Lord sends to us.

that the phone call gave her the vision to start the National Abstinence Clearinghouse to keep track of legitimate abstinence education programs (vs. those that were called abstinence but, in fact, taught "comprehensive" sex education that promoted all types of birth control). The Clearinghouse became a major player in abstinence education throughout the country and around the world.

Meanwhile, also in the 1980s, there was a growing recognition that abortion not only killed unborn babies but also had devastating effects on their mothers. The very first woman I had ever met who had had an abortion was a woman who came to volunteer at Columbus Right to Life in about 1975. She

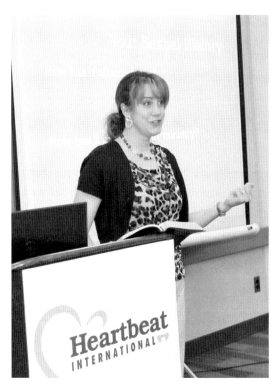

▲ *Katy Flood, Heartbeat consultant, trains leaders at a Heartbeat International conference on the concept of Sexual Integrity™ and how to implement this unique program on the local level.*

would do anything she could, she said, to help prevent other women from making an abortion decision. I was stunned by her story and her emotional state. She seemed very nervous at all times. She told me that she had been a successful attorney, contentedly married, when she discovered she had an unplanned pregnancy. Her husband told her he would leave her if she did not have an abortion. Her mother took her to the abortion clinic. When she experienced emotional "complications," her husband left her, and she could not forgive "my own mother" for assisting in the abortion. It became obvious to me for the first time that abortion affected women deeply. Soon I came to realize that it also affected men, marriage, and all family relationships.

It is hard to imagine now, with the proliferation of research on the effect of abortion, but no one had yet recognized the existence of what, in the 1990s, came to be called "post-abortion syndrome" (a form of post-traumatic stress syndrome). This condition is still not recognized by secular counseling professionals. I still regret that no one, in 1975, knew how to help this victim of abortion who came forward into the pro-life movement. She told her story publicly, and was even featured in a very early pro-life educational film, but she soon disappeared. I often think about her and pray for her, hoping that she finally found the hope and healing so available now for all those who have been involved in abortion.

By the 1980s, when I was regularly attending AAI Academies, pregnancy centers were sharing that some volunteers were entering our movement who had had abortions. Healing programs were needed, and none existed within our centers at that time. There were no professional counselors doing post-abortion counseling, at least that we could find. Our Pregnancy Distress Center in Columbus launched a post-abortion recovery program in 1984, developed by volunteers within our center who had had abortions and based on the work being done in Cincinnati through WEBA, Women Exploited by Abortion, the first post-abortion organization, I believe, in the country. This center allowed Heartbeat International to take WEBA's groundbreaking program around the world. Based on a support group model that can also be used one-on-one, the program takes a woman (or man) through the process of grieving the loss of the child, into forgiveness from the Lord, and then into commemoration of the child that was lost to abortion. It is now called *H.E.A.R.T., Healing the Effects of Abortion Related Trauma*, and it is used by Heartbeat affiliates worldwide. Happily, today, there are many excellent abortion recovery programs, and many of them have grown out of our movement.

So, by the time I became president of Heartbeat International in 1993, our pregnancy help movement encompassed programs of prevention (abstinence education), crisis intervention (pregnancy testing and counseling), support (material aid and classes in nutrition, parenting, fatherhood, and more, plus host homes and maternity homes), and healing (abortion recovery). We were clearly about more than "just" alternatives to abortion, even about more than "saving" babies and mothers from abortion. But what was the "core" that held us together and that was the explanation for our unity amidst all the diversity?

In 1994, when we published the first edition of *The LOVE Approach™*, I touched on this core in the V step, Vision and Value step, of that training manual. I wrote then that the V step involved helping the client to see that she is a child of God, loved and redeemed by Him; she is not meant for the kind of life she has been leading.

In the new edition of *The LOVE Approach*, the new vision that can and should be shared with our clients is greatly expanded. It took several years for Heartbeat to develop what I believe God was showing us to be the core of our unique opportunity in the pregnancy movement—to introduce to women a new vision of who they have been created to be by God, as female, as women, to understand their gift of femininity, especially their gift of fertility that is so endangered by the lifestyle they are leading. Once they understand and grasp the true nature of their femininity, not only will their own lives be transformed, but also these women will help rebuild the family that has been so damaged over the last forty years.

The most comprehensive explanation of this vision of true femininity in Heartbeat resources today is our Sexual Integrity™ Program. This contains materials ("a tool kit" including videos, brochures, workbooks) that can be used in our centers with "negative test" clients but also with every client, because each one needs to grasp who she was created to be as a woman. The program teaches women working in our centers, our foot soldiers, how to teach other women about sexual integrity, or sexual wholeness: emotional, intellectual, physical, social, and spiritual. This means expressing the gift of sexuality throughout life in a true, excellent, honest, and pure way. It is protection in childhood, direction in adolescence, and celebration in adulthood. It is based on several Biblical pillars from the Old and New Testaments.

The primary Biblical teachings on which the program is based are, first, Genesis 1:27–28: "God created man in his image; in the divine image he created him; male and female he created them, saying 'Be fruitful and multiply; fill the earth and subdue it'" (NAB); and, second, Ephesians 5:31–33: "'For this reason a man shall leave father and mother and be joined to his wife, and the two shall become one flesh.' This is a great mystery, but I speak in reference to Christ and the church. In any case, each one of you should love his wife as himself, and the wife should respect her husband" (ESV).

The sexual integrity message is much more complete than abstinence, which is limited to not doing something. Sexual integrity is a way of life, based on our identity as created by God, male and female, made in His image, and intended by Him to be joined together in love, cooperating with God in bringing His creation, the next generation, into the world.

In 2000, I met Carrie Abbott, a well-known abstinence educator, at one time associated with the pregnancy center in Seattle, Washington, now the head of the Legacy Institute. She and I discovered that we both had the same burden—to bring a more complete message on sexual purity to the women we served—and we began to share our own deepening understanding of what I call "God's plan for our sexuality." I was able to secure a grant from the Gerard Health Foundation to develop a comprehensive program called Sexual Integrity, and Carrie began even more intentionally to explore the subject, learning everything she could from Evangelical sources and from Catholic ones. Catholics, especially, have been leaders in this issue, and Carrie, a strong Evangelical Christian, took courses from Pope Paul VI Institute in Omaha, Nebraska, and studied *The Theology of the Body* from John Paul II. Carrie and I frequently discussed what she was learning, and, as she developed teaching ideas, she tested them in various pregnancy help centers.

Out of all this, Heartbeat's Sexual Integrity Program was first published in 2002 (and revised in 2007). It is the only program of its kind, designed specifically to help women who have come into pregnancy help centers (most of whom are deeply wounded by broken sexual relationships, abortion, and often sexual abuse) to grasp and begin to live by a new vision of themselves as created in the image and likeness of God, with a special feminine nature and gifting. (This special gifting is called the "feminine genius" by John Paul II in his inspiring Apostolic Letter, published in 1988, called "The Dignity of Women" or *Mulieris Dignitatem*, which I discovered around 1990, and which had helped shape my thinking at that time.)

One of the key "tools" in the Sexual Integrity "tool box" for use in centers and clinics, and most unique element of the program, is called *Focus on Fertility*. With a video set and workbook, it is used to teach girls and women about the beauty of how their bodies are made, and what a gift their fertility is. Instead of a curse, their monthly cycle is a gift. They can learn how to chart their cycle and understand the complexity of their reproductive system, not with a goal of avoiding sexual intimacy in the fertile time of the month, but rather with a goal of appreciating how "beautifully and wonderfully made" they are, and how important it is to protect their gift of fertility from disease and injury. This hands on approach is much more effective in changing their perception of themselves than simply telling them about their bodies or showing pictures or diagrams. Once a woman experiences the wonder of her own body and how it is designed, she has a whole new concept of how special she is as a woman, and that she deserves to be treated with respect.

As common sense as this sounds now, there was a risk to developing the program and introducing it ten years ago. Some of the concepts had been taught in Catholic circles, but would Evangelicals in our movement accept them? They have! Some proponents of teaching a hands-on approach to understanding a woman's fertility (those involved in certain Natural Family Planning programs) believe that teaching this information to unmarried women will lead to more promiscuity. Would our program come under attack for this reason? It has not! In fact, more and more people now understand that, done properly, this kind of education results in outcomes such as women leaving cohabiting relationships and choosing abstinence until marriage.

I remember my nervousness and prayers for courage when I decided that I was supposed to make the message of "God's Plan for Our Sexuality" the subject of my keynote address to the Heartbeat International Conference in 1999, and share with our affiliates that I believed that this was the deeper core that brought us all together, the message that we were all called to share with those the Lord was entrusting to us. I defined "God's Plan for Our Sexuality" as this: there are five things that in God's Plan must be together: sexual intimacy, marriage between a man and a woman, children, unconditional or selfless love, and God.

If we remove one of these from God's equation, we have most of the social ills of our time. For example, marriage without unconditional love, God, and often without children leads to loveless, Godless, material-driven partnerships that easily end in divorce. Sexual intimacy without marriage leads to cohabitation, fatherlessness, and children raised in one-parent families with all the attendant problems for those children. Sexual intimacy without selfless love and marriage leads to STIs, STDs, promiscuity, prostitution, human trafficking, and objectifying of people. Same-sex intimacy leads to the myriad of problems associated with homosexuality. Sexual intimacy without children leads to abortion, post-abortion trauma, lack of trust between men and women, and broken relationships. In fact, if you think about it, most social and personal problems today can be traced to not living out God's plan for sexuality and trying to cover the pain that results with drugs, alcohol, and other destructive behaviors.

I intended to share my belief, in this keynote, that this is the deepest core of our call in the pregnancy help movement—not only to save babies and women from abortion, but also to share this vision of God's plan for sexuality whenever we can. The core or root where all of the diverse groups and programs in the pregnancy help movement (prevention, crisis intervention, support, healing) are united is right here, God's plan for sexuality. God is using all of us to help put that plan back in place, to reconstitute it in this world today where it has almost been destroyed by the devil, through the destruction of our sexual mores. (Abortion is the linchpin because it guarantees that children can be eliminated from God's plan.)

Would this message at the conference ring true for both Catholics and Evangelicals? It did! As I spoke, I had eye contact with many people in the audience of several hundred, and I could see that they accepted what I was saying! Moreover, the Sexual Integrity Program that embodies these ideas, and provides the tools of teaching these concepts to our clients, has since been widely accepted in all types of centers and around the world.

Heartbeat's vision is that we can take this even further. The sexual integrity concepts and program tools can be combined within the medical model, or pregnancy help medical clinic, to provide true health care for women. The term "reproductive health care" as used today is simply a code term for contraceptives and abortion, neither of which leads to reproduction (their purpose is the opposite) nor to good health (in fact, there are many documented detrimental health effects associated with both contraceptives and abortion). True women's health care protects and enhances a woman's gift of fertility.

Pregnancy help medical clinics could, Heartbeat believes, eclipse Planned Parenthood (the main provider of "reproductive health care" for women, that is, contraception and abortion) and become the leading providers of true women's health care. We have been promoting that vision for about ten years. Two articles I have written discussing this vision are included in the medical manual that Heartbeat co-published several years ago with Care Net, *Medical Perspectives*. The articles are "The Fertility Frontier" and "Working with the Whole Woman."

Some of our entrepreneurial affiliates have been experimenting with various models that incorporate sexual integrity education along with fertility appreciation and even some fertility care into their services. STD testing, in particular, is a medical service provided by many of our medical clinics that opens the door to follow-up services that focus on true women's health. Some of our affiliates that have been in the forefront of these experimental programs are Elizabeth's New Life Center in Dayton, Ohio; First Way Pregnancy Support Center in Phoenix, Arizona; FirstChoice Clinic in Fargo, North Dakota; Life Center of Long Island, New York; and Birthchoice Clinics of Orange County, California.

One hundred percent pro-life medical practices are emerging in a few states, headed by heroic physicians who feel compelled to leave the standard practice of OB-GYN, dominated as it is by this ungodly view of "reproductive health care." Our pregnancy help centers and these clinics are partnering wherever possible so our clients can experience true women's health care. The model for these faith-based health care clinics is Tepeyac Family Center in Fairfax, Virginia, founded by Dr. John Bruchalski, now staffed by six physicians and a nurse practitioner.

This year, there have been major efforts in the United States to defund the major purveyor of so-called "reproductive health care" in the United States, Planned Parenthood. In the United States today, Planned Parenthood receives about $1 million per day in tax dollars through Title X for "family planning" or contraceptive services, and it provides about one-fourth of all abortions in the United States in its abortion clinics. Heartbeat stands ready to help our affiliates, partnering with the pro-life medical community, to fill the void that will be left when this Goliath falls.

Looking to the Future

What or who else is commemorating forty years of history at the same time as Heartbeat International? Well, for one, Starbucks! It was not the Holy Spirit, I would say, but rather the right vision for the right time plus good business and marketing skills that created this icon of American companies. For another, Title X, the tax-funded birth control program created by law in 1971, is also forty years old.

I don't believe it is a coincidence that Heartbeat's fortieth anniversary corresponds to that of Title X. It seems to me that God inspired great good in His church (the founding of the pregnancy help movement) to counter the great evil that was being unleashed through Title X. This program, and the new Office of Population Affairs at the U.S. Department of Health and Human Services that administers it, was promoted and lobbied for by the same people and organizations that were the masterminds of legalizing abortion on demand, all led by Planned Parenthood. They "sold" Congress and the administration on the idea that such a program was needed, based on dire predictions of a population explosion (that proved to be false), asserting that if free contraceptives were provided to "those who want them," there would be a reduction in "unwanted and untimely childbearing."

It is not my purpose to analyze the negative effects of Title X in statistical detail. That has been done very

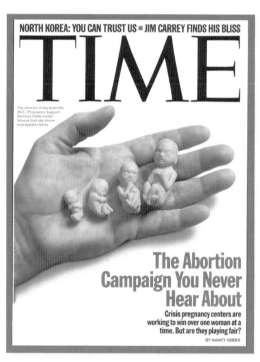

▲ Pregnancy centers and medical clinics have recently received some positive national attention, as evidenced in this TIME magazine cover story in 2007. While the reporter aimed at objectivity, and introduced TIME's millions of readers to Heartbeat International and Option Line, the magazine also included charges that our centers may not be "playing fair."

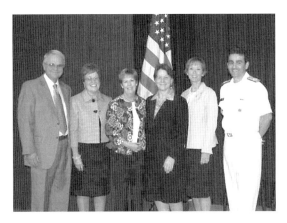

▲ *About forty thousand volunteers are involved in the pregnancy help movement in the United States, making us one of the greatest volunteer movements in our country. More than one hundred of these volunteers were honored with the President's Volunteer Award at a grand ceremony in Washington, D.C., in 2008, given by Joxel Garcia, Assistant Secretary of Health and Human Services. Pictured, L to R: Kent Underwood, Jane Underwood, Cathy Smith, Peggy Hartshorn, Linda Augspurger, and Joxel Garcia. Kent, Jane, Cathy, and Linda from Pregnancy Decision Health Center in Columbus, Ohio, received the award.*

thoroughly by others, in particular by Robert Patterson in an article entitled "Forty Years of Title X Is Enough: The Folly of the McNamara Approach to Family Planning," published in the Fall 2010 edition of the journal *The Family In America.* Two points selected from that excellent article show some of that folly: Title X has spent an inflation-adjusted $12.4 billion, yet here are some of the results: 10.7 percent of all births were to unmarried women in 1970; now that figure is 41 percent overall. It is up from 34.9 percent in the African American population in 1970 to 72.8 percent now; and among teenagers from 29.5 percent to 87.2 percent now. Does this sound like a reduction in untimely childbearing?

Title X, by promoting and funding the false view of "reproductive health" for forty years in our country, is in large part responsible for the erosion of true sexual health in this country, for the epidemic of sexually transmitted diseases, the decline of marriage and the traditional family, and for abortion on demand. Since contraceptives themselves often lead to "unplanned pregnancies," the need for and rationale for abortion increases, as do the numbers of abortions.

Title X can be seen as shorthand for a mentality that is the total opposite of sexual integrity or God's plan for sexuality that I believe is at the core of the pregnancy help movement (see chapter 13). I was amazed when, in researching Heartbeat history, I discovered that our founder Dr. John Hillabrand testified in Congress against the family planning legislation that created Title X. In his testimony, he challenged Congress to think through how easily a program that was supposed to be "voluntary" could be used to coerce especially the poor and minorities to intentionally reduce their numbers (he was so right!), and he warned that it could lead to abortions (right again!). He noted that he was a great proponent of "family planning," that is, the planning and spacing of children within the family. He was a proponent of Natural Family Planning. But, he pointed out, the term "family planning" was not defined in the legislation, and it appeared that the main goal was to prevent live births, which could also include abortions (right again!). Based on Dr. Hillabrand's testimony, the language of Title X was tightened up to make sure the funding did not pay for abortion as a means of family planning, but we are still fighting today to try to get Title X funding taken away from its major recipient, Planned Parenthood, the nation's largest abortion provider.

Dr. Hillabrand eloquently reminded Congress of the danger that their actions could potentially lead to abortion:

> *Human life, if it is at all important in our time, must be defended across the board. Any arbitrary exceptions, especially when they become legalized, are potentially dangerous to us all. The most terrible pages of history are those which tell of regimes founded on, or at least tolerant of, disregard of the intrinsic values of human life. The most glorious and courageous are those which recite the contrary. No society or civilization, in the better sense, has survived inhuman principles. Adding abortion through government policy or inadvertent permissiveness to the present state of national and international unrest would suggest little optimism for the survival of our society as we have known it.*

About six months after Dr. John's testimony, Title X was passed. That same year, Dr. John, Lore Maier, Sister Paula, and others founded AAI, now Heartbeat International. At the same time that the seeds of great evil were being sown, so were the seeds of great good.

The condition of the family has greatly deteriorated in American over the last forty years. It seems prescient that our founders chose as the AAI logo the three Hearts of Gold: two larger hearts representing the mother and father (with some markings showing the effects of maturity and experience) surrounding the tiny pure heart in the center representing the child, the "nucleus of the family," as our early literature describes it (see page 26 for logo). Again, our logo shows that our founders were not only concerned about the baby, and not only about mother and baby, but about the family as God intended it to be, and about the family as the basis for a stable society. This remained our logo until I became president of Heartbeat in 1993, but I made a point of incorporating the Hearts of Gold into our new logo. The Hearts of Gold image is the centerpiece design of our Heartbeat International Legacy Award, inaugurated at our fortieth anniversary celebration. Heartbeat International today carries this value forward.

In the last few years, pregnancy help centers and the work of Heartbeat International have gained increasing recognition within the pro-life/pro-family movement and even within the culture at large. *Time* magazine featured a surprisingly objective story on pregnancy help centers in 2007, and introduced centers and Option Line to millions of readers. Family Research Council published an excellent research report at the end of 2009, *A Passion to Serve, A Vision for Life* (available on the Heartbeat International website). It highlights many Heartbeat International affiliates and especially the services provided in centers and clinics around the country that enhance maternal and child health. These include programs that provide pregnancy support and education, parenting skills, fatherhood programs, pregnancy confirmation and early prenatal

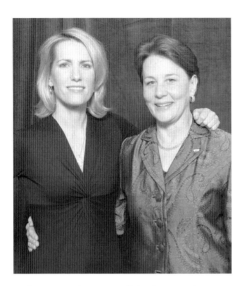

▲ Peggy receives one of the inaugural Life Prizes, given by the Gerard Health Foundation, in 2008. Laura Ingraham was the Master of Ceremonies for the gathering, held in Washington, D.C., in conjunction with the March for Life and the national conference of Students for Life. One of the goals of Ray and Marilyn Ruddy in bestowing the award is to inspire young people in the pro-life movement.

care, one-on-one support programs, referrals to important community services, and more—all of which result in healthier mothers and babies. These programs not only save lives, but they also save taxpayer dollars that need not be spent for costly care of low-birth-weight babies. By deterring abortions, our centers also save precious health care dollars that need not be spent on potential physical effects of abortion (such as problems in future pregnancies, premature births, or infertility) or potential emotional effects (such as depression, drug and alcohol abuse, and more).

Another recognition of the work of our pregnancy centers was the honor I received in being chosen for one of the first Life Prizes awards in 2008, given by the Gerard Health Foundation, a private foundation of Raymond B. and Marilyn A. Ruddy. The prizes are described this way by the Foundation on its website (www.lifeprizes.org):

Life Prizes is a prize program awarding up to $600,000 for outstanding efforts to awaken the conscience of America to the sanctity of human life through public advocacy, scientific research, outreach and public disclosure activities, legal action and other noteworthy achievements. The purpose of Life Prizes is two-fold: to recognize those on the front lines of the greatest human rights battle of our day, and to encourage and inspire the next generation to accomplish great things for the cause of life.

I considered the award to be not for myself personally, but for all the foot soldiers who are "on the front lines of the greatest human rights battle of our day." It was an honor to represent them, and perhaps even you, if you are part of this great movement through the giving of your time, talent, or treasure, or perhaps by your prayer partnership. You are helping in these ways to reach and rescue as many lives as possible through our life-affirming network of care, thus renewing communities for life. Thank you, if you are among these foot soldiers or are supporting them in your own way. The Life Prize honor is for you too! I truly hope that this great awards program serves the purpose for which it is intended: to "inspire the next generation to accomplish great things for the cause of life" and to carry the torch that this first generation is passing on.

Forty years is sometimes considered the end of a generation, especially in Biblical terms. Surely, the generation that has been involved in the first forty years of Heartbeat International history has made a tremendous difference in the lives of millions of people. A partial list of these warriors is included in appendix II, and many others are mentioned throughout this history. A whole "generation" of people are alive today primarily as a result of the first generation of foot soldiers armed with love.

Those who have gone before us in this first forty years, and those who are working with us now, are inspirational—they are like that "great cloud of witnesses" that St. Paul writes about as he remembers the stories of Gideon, Barak, Samson, David, Samuel, the prophets, and others who suffered and died for their faith, even before the coming of the Lord. St. Paul says, "Therefore, since we are surrounded by such a great cloud of witnesses, let us throw off everything that hinders and the sin that so easily entangles, and let us run with perseverance the race marked out for us" (Heb. 12:1, NIV).

In the Bible, forty days or years is seen as a time of trial, testing, or probation. It rained for forty days and forty nights. Moses was on the mountain for forty days. The Israelites wandered for forty years in the desert, Jesus fasted in the wilderness for forty days, and He was seen on earth for forty days after His resurrection until He ascended into heaven. That period of time is always followed by restoration, revival, or renewal. Heartbeat's first forty years has been a period in which our faith has been tested, and as we have trusted the Lord, He has provided, built our faith, and made it even stronger. I hope that this history properly demonstrates His faithfulness and goodness.

Almost everything seems to have changed in the last forty years. We have reflected on the sad and dramatic decline of the family due, in great part, to the fact that God's plan for sexuality is not being lived out. Yet, we have seen how God has lifted up an army of foot soldiers to contend with the enemy. While our families and family values are declining, technology, on the other hand, is advancing. Witness the new generation of pregnancy help centers and medical clinics that we have today. Forty years ago, a pregnancy center in the United States consisted of a room for counseling, a phone, and a bathroom (sometimes down the hall), needed to collect the sample for the pregnancy test. Now, modern pregnancy help medical clinics in the United States often have a high-tech ultrasound machine, additional medical technology for STD testing and treatment, and, in the business office, computers for client record keeping, accounting, and fundraising, and Internet technology for instant communication and social networking. Who would have thought of all this forty years ago?

It is almost impossible to predict what the future holds for the next generation that will move our pregnancy help movement forward. Some things, however, do not change, and these must be the basis for the advancement of Heartbeat International in the next forty years. The three things are God, human nature, and the church as the Body of Christ in this world.

First, we must continue to honor God in everything we do. We must know, love, and serve Him, and, as individual foot soldiers, we must be in relationship with Him. He is truly the General

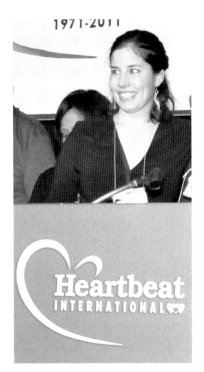

1971-2011

Heartbeat
INTERNATIONAL

▲ The next generation is being prepared to take leadership, and this was recognized when Salvadora Keith, executive director of Life Outreach Center in Houghton, Michigan, was selected to represent her peers and receive the Next Generation Legacy Award at the Heartbeat International Fortieth Anniversary Conference in 2011.

who leads and guides us all. It is His plan that we try to discern and then get on board with His plan (not set our own direction and ask Him to bless it!). He is the Alpha and the Omega. He will always provide, and His grace will be sufficient. We must seek first His kingdom, and everything else will be added on.

Second, we must recognize the truth of human nature as God created us to be. We are creatures of relationship, made in the image of God, who is a God of relationship (Father, Son, and Holy Spirit). We are male and female, and God commanded us to increase and multiply and fill the earth. What a great gift our fertility is, as God uses us to bring His most special creations into the world. We must honor the dignity of the person, as God created man and woman to be, both in our day-to-day dealings with one another, and especially with the people whom God sends us, the women and families who come into our centers, clinics, maternity homes, and other programs. We must deal with the whole person, using something like *The LOVE Approach* (perhaps by another name). We must always listen with respect, provide life-giving options, and speak the vision and value of human dignity, plus hope and healing through the Lord. And we must be ready with practical help and support, like the Good Samaritan. We must especially speak the value of the dignity of women.

Third, we must challenge the church to be the church, the Body of Christ in this world. This is the mission Jesus gave the church, so that will never change. Christians are His hands and His feet; they bring Him into a hurting and suffering world. They speak His truth into a world hungering and thirsting for it. If the church would rise up and be the church, we would not have abortion on demand in this country or around the globe.

We were reminded of this in a powerful way recently by Dr. Bernard Nathanson, one of the founders of the National Abortion Rights Action League, the partner of Planned Parenthood that led the effort to make abortion legal, resulting in the Supreme Court decision of January 22, 1973. Dr. Nathanson, an agnostic at the time, ran what he called "the world's largest abortion clinic" in New York City. By the grace of God, he recognized the humanity of the unborn child when he began to study the technology of surgical operations on the children in the womb. He said that he began to realize he was killing what could be his own patients. Dr. Nathanson eventually became a Christian and a leader in the pro-life movement in the last years of his life. He is perhaps best known for the film he produced called *The Silent Scream*. His death is another milestone in our fortieth anniversary year.

The priest who ministered to Dr. Nathanson during his long period of illness, and gave him the last rites of the Catholic Church, recounted that at one point he asked Dr. Nathanson how he and his allies were able to so quickly change the values of the nation and bring about abortion on demand with all its attendant evils. Dr. Nathanson replied simply, "The church was asleep."

This year I had the benefit of attending the National Day of Prayer service held in Washington, D.C. I was touched especially by a prayer for our church, contained in the 30-Day Prayer Guide, a prayer that the church will re-awake, that it will be on fire like the early church, that it will be overflowing with foot soldiers armed with love. It starts with a quote from James (1:27, NIV), "Religion that God our Father accepts as pure and faultless is this: to look after orphans and widows in their distress and to keep oneself from being polluted by the world." The prayer's reflection on this verse is this, and it is a fitting close:

> *Lord, the first chapters of the Book of Acts provide a reflection of the loving, healing community that the Church is meant to be, so much so that "there were no needy persons among them." I want to reach out and touch others with Your love. It might take a miracle, but help me to extend myself to my neighbors, across cultural, racial, and Church barriers. I confess that I can't do this on my own, but that You can change me through the power of Your Holy Spirit. Father, breathe life into Your Church so that it can be written that there are no needy persons among us. The need is overwhelming, but Your grace and ability to provide is greater. Revive our hearts to rise up and give and give and give. May we reflect You to a dying world, Lord Jesus, and love as You love. Amen.*

Appendix I: Heartbeat International Servant Leaders, 1996–2011

Since our twenty-fifth anniversary year, Servant Leader awards have been given annually at the Heartbeat International Conference to leaders within Heartbeat International and the broader pro-life movement. "A servant leader is one who has a servant's heart and mind, a servant's values and attitudes, but a leader's skills, a leader's vision and ingenuity, and a leader's creativity…Jesus was the greatest leader of all time…Yet Jesus had a servant's compassion." Tim Hansel

2011
Cindi Boston, Pregnancy Care Center, Springfield, MO
Lola French, Canadian Association of Pregnancy Support Services, Alberta, Canada
Elaine Ham, Pregnancy Resource Ministries, Alpharetta, GA
Patricia Lindley, National Memorial for the Unborn, Choices Pregnancy Resource Center, Chattanooga, TN

2010
Charles and Barbara Thomas, N. Baton Rouge Women's Help Center, Baton Rouge, LA
Marianne Casagranda, New Hope Pregnancy Center, Butte, MT
Sandy Epperson, Center for Pregnancy, Orlando, FL
Jorge Serrano, Centro de Ayuda para Mujer (C.A.M.), Mexico City, Mexico

2009
Pauline and George Economon, First Choice Clinic, Fargo, ND
Janet Trenda, Heartbeat International Board, Rancho Santa Margarita, CA
John Tabor, Crisis Pregnancy Center of Tucson, Tucson, AZ
Dr. Levon Yuille, The Bible Church, Ypsilanti, MI

2008
Dr. Alveda King, King for America, Atlanta, GA
Pat Layton, A Woman's Place, Tampa, FL
Edward and Barbra Mwansa, Silent Voices, Kitwe, Zambia
Julie Parton, Ph.D., Texas Life Connection, Dallas, TX

2007
Anne Foster, Pregnancy Help Australia (P.H.A.), Canberra, Australia
Sam and Gloria Lee, Campaign Life Missouri, St. Louis, MO
Dinah Monahan, Hope House Maternity Home, Show Low, AZ

2006
Russ Amerling, Choose Life Inc., Ocala, FL
Linda Augspurger, Pregnancy Decision Health Centers, Columbus, OH
Beth Diemert, LifeSteward Ministries, Knoxville, TN

2005
Kelle Berry, Option Line, Columbus, OH
Susan Brown, PregnancyCare of Cincinnati, Cincinnati, OH
Vicky Botsford McCarter, LifeSteward Ministries, Nashville, TN
Father Frank Pavone, Priests for Life, Staten Island, NY

2004

Kurt Entsminger, J.D., Care Net, Lansdowne, PA

Vivian Koob, Elizabeth's New Life Center, Dayton, OH

Gail Schreiner, Africa Cares for Life, Seadoone, NL South Africa

2003

Rev. David Bentley, Mission to Ukraine, Zhitomir, Ukraine

Eric Keroack, M.D., A Woman's Concern, Boston, MA

Mary Suarez-Hamm, Centro Tepeyac, Silver Spring, MD

John C. Willke, M.D., Life Issues Institute, Cincinnati, OH

2002

Dr. Elaine Eng, Boro Pregnancy Counseling Center, Bayside, NY

Olusegun Famure, Nigeria Life League, Nigeria

Thomas Glessner, J.D., NIFLA, Fredericksburg, VA

Mike Hartshorn, J.D., Heartbeat International Board, Columbus, OH

2001

Sheila Boyle, Crisis Pregnancy Center, Bethel Park, PA

Kurt Dillinger, Life International, Grand Rapids, MI

Rev. Johnny and Pat Hunter, LEARN, Fayetteville, NC

Bethany Woodcock, Hope for Life, Greece

2000

Jim Manning, Project REACH, New York, NY

Juergen Severloh, The Family Support Center, Winnipeg, Canada

Julie Wilson, Teller Pregnancy Resource Center, Woodland Park, CO

Rev. Curtis Young, Church of the Atonement, Silver Spring, MD

1999

Molly Kelly, Pennsylvanians for Human Life, Horsham, PA

Pat Lassen, Pregnancy Services of Gratiot County, Alma, MI

Imre Teglasy, ALFA Alliance, Budapest, Hungary

1998

Rev. John Ensor, A Woman's Concern, Boston, MA

Pamela Smith, M.D., Lawndale Christian Health Center, Chicago, IL

1997

Carol Aronis, PregnancyCare of Cincinnati, Cincinnati, OH

Margaret Lee, Orlando, FL

1996

Esther Applegate, A.A.I. Consultant, Toledo, OH

Alice and Frank Brown, M.D., A.A.I. Board, St. Cloud, MN

John Hillabrand, M.D., A.A.I. Board, Toledo, OH (posthumous)

Annette Krycinski, A.A.I. Board, Dimondale, MI

Lore Maier, A.A.I. Executive Director, Toledo, OH

Anne and Jimmy Pierson, Loving and Caring, Lancaster, PA

Ursula and Ed Slaggert, Abortion Alternatives Information Inc., Saginaw, MI

Marilyn Szewczyk, A.A.I. Board, Baltimore, MD

Sister Paula Vandegaer, A.A.I. Board, International Life Services, Los Angeles, CA

Dr. Margaret White, A.A.I. Board, Croyden, England

Mary Winter, A.A.I. Board, Pittsburgh, PA

Appendix II: Longtime Foot Soldiers

The following foot soldiers are recognized here for their many years of active duty in the Compassion arm of the pro-life movement worldwide. Each has served for at least one decade, and many for two or three decades. They are listed with the pregnancy help ministry where they started their leadership service (as founders, board leaders, or staff leaders), but some have moved into positions with other organizations, some into national leadership. A few have passed on to their eternal reward. Their organizations have been affiliated with Heartbeat International, and Heartbeat International knows these warriors personally.

We realize that we may have inadvertently omitted some here that should have been included, but that risk was overshadowed by the greater value of recognizing so many outstanding foot soldiers. Please let us know the names of others who should be included in this list.

Carrie Abbott, Life Choices of King County, Seattle, WA
Nile Abele, Stillwater Life Services Inc., Stillwater, OK
Karen Abott, The Pregnancy Center, Clinton, IA
Kathie Archer, Crisis Pregnancy Center of Central AR, North Little Rock, AR
Catherine Arnsperger, Loving Choices Pregnancy Centers of NW AR, Rogers, AR
Carol Aronis, Pregnancy Care Center, Cincinnati, OH
Linda Augspurger, Pregnancy Decision Health Centers, Columbus, OH
Kimberly Banks, First Choice Pregnancy Center, Texarkana, TX
Lucia Barone, Collier Pregnancy Center, Naples, FL
Barbara Beavers, Center for Pregnancy Choices Metro, Jackson, MS
Linda Bertolami, Pregnancy Choices Clinic, Union City, CA
Karen Boots, Choices Pregnancy Center, Redwood Falls, MN
Cindi Boston, Pregnancy Care Center, Springfield, MO
Sheila Boyle, Pregnancy Resource Center of South Hills, Bethel Park, PA
Kathy Bozyk, Southside Pregnancy Center, Oak Lawn, IL
Rindy Brooks, Heartbeats of Licking County, Newark, OH
Laura Buddenburg, Essential Pregnancy Services, Omaha, NE
Marianne Casagranda, New Hope Pregnancy Clinic, Butte, MT
Beth Chase, Life Choices of King County, Seattle, WA
Joanne Coker, Heart and Hands Pregnancy Care Center, Aberdeen, WA
Kim Conroy, Life Choices, Joplin, MO
Will Cossairt, Total Life Care Centers, St. Paul, MN
Paula Cullen, Life Services of Spokane, Spokane, WA
Joe Dalton, Pregnancy Resource Center of Rolla, Rolla, MO
Arlene Davis, New Beginnings, Siloam Springs, AR
Lori DeVillez, Austin Pregnancy Resource Center, Austin, TX
Beth Diemert, Women's Choice Network, Pittsburgh, PA
Kurt Dillinger, Pregnancy Resource Center, Grand Rapids, MI
Kathleen Eaton, Birth Choice, Santa Ana, CA
Pauline Economon, First Choice Clinic, Fargo, ND
Dr. Elaine Eng, The Boro Pregnancy Center, Bayside, NY
John Ensor, A Woman's Concern, Boston, MA
Sandy Epperson, First Life Center for Pregnancy, Orlando, FL
Dave and Joanne Everitt, CPCs of Greater Phoenix, Phoenix, AZ
Vonetta Ferguson, Pregnancy Help Center, Wichita Falls, TX
Vicky Filiatreau, Laurel County Life Center, London, KY
Katy Flood, Crossroads Pregnancy Center, Lewistown, PA
Nancy Foral, Essential Pregnancy Services, Omaha, NE
Susan Gallucci, Northwest Center, Washington, DC
Lorraine Gariboldi, AAA Pregnancy Options, Deer Park, NY
Kaye Gauder, Akron Pregnancy Services, Akron, OH

Jor-El Godsey, Hope Women's Center of Broward County, Davie, FL
Ellen Golias, Heartbeat of Ottawa County, Port Clinton, OH
Cookie Gray, LifeCare of Brandon, Brandon, FL
Paula Grimsley, Alpha Center, Fort Collins, CO
Kimberly Hackett-Schmidt, With Child, Phoenix, AZ
Alexis Hale, Caring for Miami, Miami, FL
Elaine Ham, Piedmont Women's Center, Greenville, SC
Virginia Hickey, AIM Women's Center and Clinic, Steubenville, OH
Merridy Hoover, Heartbeats of Licking County, Newark, OH
Margaret Horvath, Heartbeat of Monroe, Monroe, MI
Lisa Hosler, Susquehanna Valley Pregnancy Services, Lebanon, PA
Prudence Humber, Alpha Pregnancy Services, Philadelphia, PA
Becky Hyde, Arlington Pregnancy Center, Arlington, TX
Sallie Janowiak, Matrix Pregnancy Resource Center, Lafayette, IN
Sylvia Johnson, Fifth Ward Pregnancy Help Center, Houston, TX
Amy Jones, Christian Life Home, Raleigh, NC
Janet Kimes, Women's Care Center, Parkersburg, WV
Beverly Kline, Living Alternatives, Tyler, TX
Nancy Knowlton, Cookeville Pregnancy Clinic, Cookeville, TN
Vivian Koob, Elizabeth's New Life Center, Dayton, OH
Jeanette Kuiphof, Whittier Pregnancy Care Center, Whittier, CA
Pat Lassen, Pregnancy Services of Gratiot County, Alma, MI
Patricia Layton, A Woman's Place Ministries Inc., Tampa, FL
Gloria Lee, Our Lady's Inn, St. Louis, MO
Nancy Lincoln, Open Arms Pregnancy Center, DeWitt, IA
Pat Lindley, Choices Pregnancy Resource Center, Chattanooga, TN
Marsha Ludmann, Heartbeat of Columbiana County, East Liverpool, OH
Linda Lueke, Cornerstone Among Women, Elyria, OH
Anne Manice, Pregnancy Help, New York, NY
Ann Manion, Women's Care Center, South Bend, IN
John Margand, Project REACH, New York City, NY
Stacy Massey, ARIN (Abortion Recovery InterNational Inc.), Irvine, CA
John McCastle, Alliance for Life Missouri, Lee's Summit, MO
John and Randi McDonnell, Birth Choice of San Marcos, San Marcos, CA
Betty McDowell, Pregnancy Decision Health Centers, Columbus, OH
Carole McMahon, Genesis of Pittsburgh, Pittsburgh, PA
Angela McNaughton, Elinor Martin Home, New Rochelle, NY
Bobbie Meyer, Pregnancy Resource Center, Charlotte, NC
Marsha Middleton, Pregnancy Support Center, Lebanon, MO
Dinah Monahan, Living Hope Women's Centers, Show Low, AZ
Rod Murphy, Problem Pregnancy of Worcester, Worcester, MA
Lenna Neill, Piedmont Women's Center, Greenville, SC

Brenda Newport, Women's Care Center, Erie, PA

Debra Neybert, Richland Pregnancy Center, Mansfield, OH

Barbara Niedermeier, Pregnancy Helpline of Janesville, Janesville, WI

Darlene Norberg, Dallas Pregnancy Resource Center, Dallas, TX

Anne O'Connor, RTL League of Southern California, Pasadena, CA

Paula Odom, Mid Cities Pregnancy Center, Richland Hills, TX

Pam Palumbo, Bowie Crofton Pregnancy Clinic, Bowie, MD

Vikki Parker, A Woman's Place Pregnancy Resource Center, Cabot, AR

Julie Parton, Prestonwood Pregnancy Center, Dallas, TX

CJ Payne, CPC Pregnancy Resources, Davenport, IA

Linda Perry, Assist Pregnancy Center, Annandale, VA

Donna Phillips, Concern for Women, Iowa City, IA

Talitha Phillips, Resource and Support Center, Los Angeles, CA

Sol Pitchon, New Life Solutions Inc., Largo, FL

Mike Reid, Pregnancy Resource Centers of Greater Portland, Portland, OR

Raul and Chris Reyes, Life Network, Colorado Springs, CO

Sheila Riely, Life Choices Women's Clinic, Phoenix, AZ

Sally Rosiek, Conejo Valley Women's Resource Center, Thousand Oaks, CA

Eleanor Ruder, The Bridge to Life, Bayside, NY

Amy Scheuring, Women's Choice Network, Pittsburgh, PA

Linda Schindler, Miami Valley Women's Center, Dayton, OH

Chris Slattery, Expectant Mother Care, New York, NY

Mattie Sparks, Heartbeat of Sandusky, Sandusky, OH

James Sprague, Pregnancy Resource Center, Grand Rapids, MI

Sherry Sprouse, Heartbeat of Fremont, Fremont, OH

Dan Steiner, Life Centers, Indianapolis, IN

Mary Suarez Hamm, Centro Tepeyac, Silver Spring Women's Center, Silver Spring, MD

John Tabor, Crisis Pregnancy Centers of Tucson, Tucson, AZ

Karen Tameling, Options Pregnancy Resource Centers, Corvallis, OR

Jill Taylor, Pregnancy Support Center of Stark County, Canton, OH

Barbara and Charles Thomas, North Baton Rouge Women's Help Center, Baton Rouge, LA

Ruth Tibstra, Southside Pregnancy Center, Oak Lawn, IL

Gail Tierney, Bowie Crofton Pregnancy Clinic, Bowie, MD

Gay Tillotson, Collage Center, Kearney, NE

Janet Trenda, Alternate Avenues, Montclair, CA

Kim Triller, Care Net Pregnancy and Family Services, Tacoma, WA

Leslee Unruh, Alpha Center, Sioux Falls, SD

Judy Van Wagner, Community Pregnancy Centers of Northwest Ohio, Bryan, OH

Kim Warburton, Pregnancy Resource Center of Metro Richmond, Richmond, VA

Terry Winship, Care Net Pregnancy and Resource Clinic, Casper, WY

Conrad Wojnar, The Women's Center, Chicago, IL

Catherine Wood, Pregnancy Decision Health Centers, Columbus, OH

Maureen Yockey, Alternatives Pregnancy Center, Central, Denver, CO

Jackie Carney, Pregnancy Center West, Cincinnati, OH

John Banda, Pregnancy Decision Health Center, Copperbelt, Zambia

Lena Batina, Kharkov Pregnancy Assistance Center, Kharkov, Ukraine

Judith Brown, Sunparlour Pregnancy Resource Centre, Leamington, ON, Canada

Diana Castillo, Gravida—Centro de Asistencia, San Pedro, BA, NA

Marea Crick, Pregnancy Support Line, Beacon Hill, NSW, Australia

Lourdes Delgado, Centro de Ayuda para la Mujer, Mexico City, Mexico

Lola French, CAPSS (Canadian Association of Pregnancy Support Services), Red Deer, AB, Canada

Marina Karavas, Hope for Life, Pireaus, Greece

Barbra and Edward Mwansa, Kitwe, Nkana, Zambia

Brian Norton, Christian Advocacy Society, Burnaby, BC, Canada

Lilly Perez, Pregnancy Services of Asia, Makati City, Philippines

Vesna Radeka, Choose Life Center, Vojvodina, Serbia

Gail Schreiner, Africa Cares for Life, Durban, South Africa

Jorge Serrano, Centro De Ayuda Para La Mujer, Anzurez, Mexico D.F., Mexico

Juergen Severloh, The Family Support Centre of Winnepeg, Winnepeg, MB, Canada

Fr. Michael Shields, Magadan Women's Consultation Center, Magadan, Russia

Imre Teglasy, ALFA Alliance, Budapest, Hungary

Cristina Valea, Pro Vita Medica Foundation, Timisoara, Romania

Theresa White, Okanagan Valley Pregnancy Care Centre, Kelowna, BC, Canada

Ruth Yeboah, Life Centre of Ghana, Adum Kumasi, Ghana

Appendix III: Heartbeat International Board Members, 1971–2011

Diane Abernathy, West Chester, OH
Barbara Williamson Adams, Dallas, TX
A. G. Ladd Alexander, Shreveport, LA
Florina Alexander, Shreveport, LA
Esther Applegate, Toledo, OH
Carol Aronis, Loveland, OH
Dr. Conrad W. Baars, San Antonio, TX
Peggy Becker, Cincinnati, OH
Fred Bein, Columbus, OH
Ann Boyle, Glasgow, Scotland
Alice Brown, St. Cloud, MN
Dr. Frank Brown, St. Cloud, MN
Judie Brown, Washington, D.C.
Dorothy Butcher, Palos Verdes, CA
Rev. Charles Patrick Carroll, Collegeville, MN
Pat Chumbley, Phoenix, AZ
John Cissel, Lynnfield, MA
Cathy Clark, Yorba Linda, CA
Msgr. Eugene V. Clark, Crestwood, NY
Ken Clark, Yorba Linda, CA
Gary Crum, Washington, D.C.
Paula Salsedo Cullen, Spokane, WA
Chris Dattilo, Sudbury, MA
Mercedes R. de Martinez, Bogota, Colombia
Pia de Solenni, Crescent City, CA
Nancy Donner, Columbus, OH
Charles Donovan, Manassas, VA
Msgr. Michael J. Doyle, Toledo, OH
Jim Dundas, Dover, DE
Grit Ebner, Vienna, Austria
Randy Engel, Export, PA
John Ensor, Boston, MA
Diana Escobar, Pensacola, FL
Maria Fitzpatrick, Phoenix, AZ
Dr. James Ford, Downey, CA
Thomas Glessner, Fredericksburg, VA
Felicia Goeken, Alton, IL
Rev. Gilberto Gomez, Bogota, Columbia
Karen Gregoire, Great Falls, MT
Marion V. Grimes, Lackawanna, NY
Rev. Richard Groshek, Lansing, MI
Thomas Hajdukiewicz, Sewickley, PA
Mari Anne Hamilton-Cotter, Chicago, IL
Mary Suarez Hamm, Silver Spring, MD
Nola Hanes, Ann Arbor, MI
Bente V. Hansen, Oslo, Norway
Jane Hanzel, Detroit, MI
John E. Harrington, Peterborough, ON, Canada
Margaret Hartshorn, Columbus, OH
Michael Hartshorn, Columbus, OH
Jackie Henry, Glen Ellyn, IL
Marie Hern, Milwaukee, WI
Dr. John Hillabrand, Todedo, OH
Mary Anne Hughes, South Bend, IN
Patricia Hunter, Fayetteville, NC
Larry Jacobs, Rockford, IL
Rosemary Hamilton Jandron, East Lansing, MI
Marie Karbus, Granada Hills, CA
Vanessa Garza Kelly, Arlington, VA
Alveda King, Atlanta, GA
Annette Krycinski, Dimondale, MI
Charles Lamar, Frisco, CO

Jeremiah Leary, Cincinnati, OH
Margaret Leary, Cincinnati, OH
Rev. Stephen Letourneau, Hayes, KS
Ceil Levatino, Las Cruces, NM
Anthony Levatino, Las Cruces, NM
Lorna Lincke, Whittier, CA
Dyxie Lincoln, Colorado Springs, CO
Gregory Loesch, Columbus, OH
Betty Loescher, Minneapolis, MN
Anthony Logan, Indianapolis, IN
Peg Luksik, Johnstown, PA
Barbara Lund, Fargo, ND
Dr. William A. Lynch, Boston, MA
Lore Maier, Toledo, OH
Jim Manning, New York, NY
Rita Marker, Snohomish, WA
Elinor Martin, Yonkers, NY
Derek McCoy, Seabrook, MD
Brandon McCrary, Dallas, TX
Anne McDonald, Fort Wayne, IN
Carol McMahon, Pittsburgh, PA
Marie Meaney, Front Royal, VA
Dr. Patricia Mena, Santiago, Chili
Ancil Mitchell, Oxnard, CA
Dr. John F. Monagle, Toledo, OH
Elizabeth Mullins, St. Louis, MO
Anne Murray, La Habra, CA
Rev. Denis O'Brien, Mexico, Mexico
Bodil B. Oftestad, Oslo, Norway
Joseph Orr, Toledo, OH
Rev. Prof. Daniel Ch. Overduin, Everard Park, S. Australia
Julie Parton, Garland, TX
Robert Pearson, Honolulu, HI
Steven J. Perrin, Wichita, KS
Judy Peterson, Orlando, FL
Anne Pierson, Lancaster, PA
Rev. Pierre Primeau, Bogota, Columbia
Sister Maryann Regensburger, Waukegan, IL
Victor G. Rosenblum, Chicago, IL
David Rudolph, Los Angeles, CA
Richard L. Schleicher, Huntington Beach, CA
Dr. Edward Sheridan, Washington, D.C.
Andy Show, Columbus, OH
Marilyn Szewczyk, Baltimore, MD
John Tabor, Tucson, AZ
Janet Trenda, Ontario, CA
Patrick Trueman, Chicago, IL
Sister Paula Vandegaer, Los Angeles, CA
Joseph G. M. Vidoli, Perrysburg, OH
John Wasserman, Toledo, OH
Mary Weyrick, Paso Robles, CA
Margaret White, Croyden, England
Grace Willett, Washington, DC
Ken Willig, Snohomish, CA
Joyce Wilson, Columbus, OH
Mary Winter, Pittsburgh, PA
Rev. Carey C. Womble, M.D., Tucson, AZ
Rev. Curtis J. Young, Washington, DC

Appendix IV: Heartbeat International Conference Host Cities, 1972–2011

2011 Columbus, OH
2010 Orlando, FL
2009 Richmond, VA
2008 Dallas, TX
2007 St. Louis, MO
2006 Orlando, FL
2005 Chicago, IL
2004 Charlotte, NC
2003 Omaha, NE
2002 Pittsburgh, PA
2001 Glendale, CA
2000 Columbus, OH
1999 Washington, DC
1998 St. Louis, MO
1997 Orlando, FL
1996 Chicago, IL
1995 Pittsburgh, PA
1994 Columbus, OH
1993 St. Paul, MN
1992 Cincinnati, OH
1991 Toledo, OH
1990 Pittsburgh, PA
1989 Lake Buena Vista, FL
1988 Detroit, MI
1987 Baltimore, MD
1986 Columbus, OH
1985 Denver, CO
1984 Baltimore, MD
1983 Lansing, MI
1982 New York, NY
1981 Phoenix, AZ
1980 Chicago, IL
1979 Washington, DC
1978 St. Louis, MO
1977 Pittsburgh, PA
1976 New Orleans, LA
1975 Los Angeles, CA
1974 Toledo, OH
1973 Kenosha, WI
1972 Collegeville, MN

Appendix V: Heartbeat International Affiliates in Fortieth Anniversary Year

Copper Basin Pregnancy Center, Glennallen, AK
Always Hope Pregnancy Center Inc., Enterprise, AL
Ann's New Life Center for Women Inc., Pell City, AL
COPE Pregnancy Center, Montgomery, AL
Her Choice Birmingham Women's Center, Birmingham, AL
Her Choice North Alabama Women's Center Inc., Hanceville, AL
Mary's Haven Pregnancy Resource Center, Prattville, AL
Sav-A-Life of Dale County Inc., Ozark, AL
Wiregrass Emergency Pregnancy Svc., Daleville, AL
A Woman's Place PRC, Cabot, AR
A Woman's Place PRC, Beebe, AR
Assemblies of God Family Services Agency, Hot Springs, AR
Concepts of Truth Inc., Wynne, AR
Crisis Pregnancy Center of Central Arkansas, North Little Rock, AR
Friends for Life, Searcy, AR
Friends for Life, Heber Springs, AR
Hannah Pregnancy Resource Center, El Dorado, AR
Hannah Pregnancy Resource Center, Magnolia, AR
Hannah Pregnancy Resource Center, Camden, AR
Heart to Heart Pregnancy Support Center Inc., Fort Smith, AR
Life Choices, Crossett, AR
Loving Choices Pregnancy Center, Fayetteville, AR
Loving Choices Pregnancy Centers of NW AR, Rogers, AR
New Beginnings Pregnancy Services, Siloam Springs, AR
Pregnancy Resource Center, Jonesboro, AR
St. Joseph's Helpers/Arkansas PRC, Little Rock, AR
1st Way of Maricopa County, Phoenix, AZ
Advice & Aid Pregnancy Center, Kingman, AZ
Crisis Pregnancy Centers, Glendale, AZ
Crisis Pregnancy Centers, Phoenix, AZ
Crisis Pregnancy Centers, Mesa, AZ
Family First Pregnancy Care Center, Oracle, AZ
Family First Pregnancy Care Center, Winkelman, AZ
Fatima Women's Center, Tucson, AZ
Hope Crisis Pregnancy Center, Flagstaff, AZ
House of Ruth Pregnancy Care Center, Cottonwood, AZ
Life Choices Women's Clinic, Phoenix, AZ
Life Connections Pregnancy Resource & Referral, Prescott, AZ
Living Hope Women's Center, Springerville, AZ
Living Hope Women's Center, Whiteriver, AZ
Living Hope Women's Centers, Show Low, AZ
New Life Pregnancy Center, Bullhead City, AZ
New Life Pregnancy Center, Casa Grande, AZ
New Life Pregnancy Center, Holbrook, AZ
New Life Pregnancy Center, St. Johns, AZ
New Life Pregnancy Center, Yuma, AZ
New Life Pregnancy Center, Florence, AZ
New Life Pregnancy Center, Phoenix, AZ
New Life Pregnancy Centers, Tucson, AZ
The Crisis Pregnancy Centers of Tucson, Tucson, AZ
The Life Resource Center, Tucson, AZ
Women's Pregnancy Center, Tucson, AZ
A Woman's Friend Pregnancy Resource Center, Marysville, CA
A Women's Care Center, Chino, CA
Alpha Pregnancy Resource Center, Vacaville, CA
Alpha Pregnancy Resource Center, Fairfield, CA
Alpha Pregnancy Resource Center, Vallejo, CA
Alternate Avenues, Montclair, CA
Alternatives Women's Center, Escondido, CA
Angels Way Maternity Home, Woodland Hills, CA
Birth Choice of Imperial Valley, El Centro, CA

Birth Choice of Oceanside, Oceanside, CA
Birth Choice of San Marcos, San Marcos, CA
Birth Choice of Temecula, Temecula, CA
Care Pregnancy Center of Tulare County, Visalia, CA
CHOICES, Women's Resource Center, Pomona, CA
College Area Pregnancy Services, San Diego, CA
Compassion Pregnancy Services, Hollister, CA
Corona Life Services, Corona, CA
Crisis Pregnancy Center, Palm Desert, CA
Fallbrook Pregnancy Resource Center, Fallbrook, CA
Foothill Pregnancy Center, Sonora, CA
Foothills Pregnancy Resource Center, Duarte, CA
Harbor Pregnancy Services, Wilmington, CA
Heart to Heart Napa Valley PSC, Napa, CA
Horizon Pregnancy Center, Huntington Beach, CA
Life Centers of Ventura County, Oxnard, CA
Life Choices Pregnancy Center, Poway, CA
Life Choices Pregnancy Clinic of Ojai Valley, Ojai, CA
Life Light Pregnancy Help Center, Redding, CA
Living Help Center, Downey, CA
LivingWell Medical Clinic, Grass Valley, CA
Lompoc Crisis Pregnancy Center Inc., Lompoc, CA
Manteca RTL Pregnancy Help Center, Manteca, CA
Mary's Shelter, Santa Ana, CA
Modesto Pregnancy Center, Modesto, CA
Nightlight Christian Adoptions, Anaheim Hills, CA
Pregnancy Care Center, Ridgecrest, CA
Pregnancy Counseling Center, Mission Hills, CA
Pregnancy Counseling Services, Placerville, CA
Pregnancy Resource Center, Vista, CA
Pregnancy Resource Center of Marin, Novato, CA
Pregnancy Resource Center–Kern River Valley, Lake Isabella, CA
Ramona Pregnancy Care Clinic, Ramona, CA
Real Hope Center, El Centro, CA
Right to Life League of Southern CA, Pasadena, CA
Sacramento Life Center, Sacramento, CA
Sacramento Life Center–Roseville, Roseville, CA
Santa Ana Life Center, Santa Ana, CA
Santee Choices Pregnancy Care Center, Santee, CA
Silent Voices, Chula Vista, CA
The San Bernardino Pregnancy Resource Center, San Bernardino, CA
Ventura County Pregnancy Center, Ventura, CA
Whittier Pregnancy Care Clinic, Whittier, CA
Women's Resource Clinic, Chico, CA
A Caring Pregnancy Center, Pueblo, CO
Alpha Center, Fort Collins, CO
Eastern Plains Women's Resource Center, Byers, CO
Family Life Services, Colorado Springs, CO
Lighthouse Resource & Pregnancy Center, Westcliffe, CO
Pagosa Pregnancy Support Center, Pagosa Springs, CO
Pregnancy Resource Center, Greeley, CO
Safe Harbor Pregnancy Resource Center, Limon, CO
Salida Pregnancy & Family Center, Salida, CO
Care Net Pregnancy Center of NE CT, Danielson, CT
Care Net Pregnancy Center of NE CT, Willimantic, CT
Carolyn's Place, Waterbury, CT
Capitol Hill Pregnancy Center, Washington, DC
Northwest Center Maternity Home, Washington, DC
Sanctuaries for Life: Birthing-n-Care Program, Washington, DC
The Northwest Center, Washington, DC
Sussex Pregnancy Care Center Inc., Georgetown, DE

A Center for Women and Life for Kids, Winter Park, FL
A Woman's Answer Medical Center, Gainesville, FL
A Woman's Choice Inc., Lakeland, FL
A Woman's Place, Tampa, FL
A Woman's Place Ministries Inc., Tampa, FL
A Women's Pregnancy Center, Tallahassee, FL
A Women's Pregnancy Center, Madison, FL
A Women's Pregnancy Center, Marianna, FL
Accept Pregnancy Center, Winter Garden, FL
Alpha Center Inc., Pensacola, FL
Alpha Pregnancy Center of Palm Coast, Palm Coast, FL
Collier Pregnancy Centers Inc., Naples, FL
Cornerstone Pregnancy Center, Orlando, FL
Crestview Pregnancy Center, Crestview, FL
First Life Center for Pregnancy, Orlando, FL
Good News for Life (Alpha Center for Women), Ocala, FL
Hannah's Hope Pregnancy Care Center, Casselberry, FL
Heartbeat of Miami, Miami, FL
Hope Pregnancy Care Center, Bushnell, FL
House of Grace Maternity Home, Lynn Haven, FL
House of Grace Maternity Home, Panama City, FL
Immokalee Pregnancy Center Inc., Immokalee, FL
JMJ Life Center, Orlando, FL
JMJ Life Center, Saint Cloud, FL
JMJ Life Center Inc., Orlando, FL
Life Choices Women's Center, Longwood, FL
LIFE Inc., Fort Walton Beach, FL
LifeCare of Brandon, Brandon, FL
LifeChoices Women's Care, Lutz, FL
Lifeline Resources Inc., Jacksonville, FL
Life's Choices of Lake County Inc., Eustis, FL
New Life Solutions Inc., Pinellas Park, FL
New Life Solutions Inc., Largo, FL
New Life Solutions Inc., Clearwater, FL
Open Door Women's Clinic, Tallahassee, FL
Options for Women Pregnancy Help Clinic, Lakeland, FL
Osceola Pregnancy Center, Kissimmee, FL
Pregnancy & Family Life Center, Inverness, FL
Pregnancy & Parenting Support Services, Spring Hill, FL
Pregnancy & Parenting Support Services, Dade City, FL
Pregnancy Care Center, Stuart, FL
Pregnancy Care Center, Lake City, FL
Pregnancy Care Center, Tampa, FL
Pregnancy Care Center, Live Oak, FL
Pregnancy Care Center Inc., Fort Pierce, FL
Pregnancy Help & Information Center, Tallahassee, FL
Pregnancy Help Medical Clinic, Hialeah, FL
Pregnancy Help Medical Clinic, North Miami, FL
Pregnancy Plus Medical, Tampa, FL
Pregnancy Plus Medical, St. Petersburg, FL
Pregnancy Resource Center of Panama City Inc., Panama City, FL
Pregnancy Resource Center of Milton, Milton, FL
Pregnancy Solutions Inc., Venice, FL
Sanford Crisis Pregnancy Center, Sanford, FL
West Pasco Pregnancy Center, New Port Richey, FL
Women's Help Center, Jacksonville, FL
Women's Help Center–Beaches, Jacksonville, FL
Women's Help Center–St. Nicholas, Jacksonville, FL
Women's Pregnancy Center, Ocala, FL
Advice & Aid Pregnancy Problem Center, Hapeville, GA
Atlanta Care Center Inc., Atlanta, GA
Atlanta Pregnancy Resource Center, Tucker, GA
Care Net Pregnancy Resource Center of Atlanta, Atlanta, GA
Choices of the Heart, Statesboro, GA
Coastal Pregnancy Center, Savannah, GA
Coweta Pregnancy Services, Newnan, GA
Dahlonega Care Center Inc., Dahlonega, GA
Options Now, Valdosta, GA

Paulding Pregnancy Services, Hiram, GA
Pregnancy Resource Center, Carrollton, GA
Pregnancy Resource Center Medical Clinic, Douglasville, GA
Pregnancy Resource Center of Henry County, McDonough, GA
Rachel's House Pregnancy Clinic, Vidalia, GA
Women's First Choice Medical, Tifton, GA
Women's Pregnancy Center, Marietta, GA
Pregnancy Problem Center of Honolulu, Honolulu, HI
The Pregnancy Center–Kona, Kailua Kona, HI
A New Beginning/Catholic Charities, Des Moines, IA
Alpha Center, Sioux City, IA
Catholic Charities, Council Bluffs, IA
Heartland Pregnancy Center, Ottumwa, IA
LifeCare Pregnancy Center, Stuart, IA
New Horizons Adoption Agency Inc., Mason City, IA
Pathways of Pella, Pella, IA
Ruth Harbor, Des Moines, IA
The Pregnancy Center, Clinton, IA
A Blessed Beginning, Bonners Ferry, ID
Clearwater Valley Pregnancy/Life Skills Center, Kamiah, ID
Hope Pregnancy Center of Central ID, Grangeville, ID
Open Arms PCC and Real Choices Clinic, Coeur d'Alene, ID
Abigail Women's Clinic, Mendota, IL
Aid for Women, Chicago, IL
Aid for Women, Berwyn, IL
Fontebella Maternity Home, O'Fallon, IL
Fox Valley Pregnancy Center, South Elgin, IL
Fox Valley Pregnancy Clinic, St. Charles, IL
Gianna's House PRC, Rock Falls, IL
Loving Arms Crisis Pregnancy Center, Taylorville, IL
River Valley Pregnancy Resource Center, Bradley, IL
Southside Pregnancy Center, Oak Lawn, IL
Waterleaf Women's Center, Aurora, IL
Woman's Choice Services, Lombard, IL
Woman's Choice Services, Downers Grove, IL
Woman's Choice Services, Hinsdale, IL
Woman's Choice Services, Crest Hill, IL
Women's Care Clinic, Danville, IL
Women's Pregnancy Center, Galesburg, IL
A Hope Center at Grabill, Grabill, IN
A Hope Center at Primetime, Fort Wayne, IN
A Hope Center Pregnancy & Relationship Resources, Fort Wayne, IN
A Hope Center Southwest, Fort Wayne, IN
Crisis Pregnancy Center of Bloomington, Bloomington, IN
Gospel of Life Pregnancy Help Center, Brookville, IN
Great Lakes Gabriel Project, Columbus, IN
Heartline Pregnancy Center, Warsaw, IN
L.I.F.E. Center, Wabash, IN
L.I.F.E. Center Inc., North Manchester, IN
Life and Family Services, Kendallville, IN
LIFE Pregnancy Help Center Inc., Paoli, IN
Matrix Pregnancy Resource Center, Lafayette, IN
Pregnancy Care Center, Lawrenceburg, IN
Pregnancy Care Center of Jay County, Portland, IN
Pregnancy Care Center of Washington Inc., Washington, IN
Pregnancy Choices, Linton, IN
Pregnancy Help Center, Marion, IN
RETA, Elkhart, IN
The Hope Clinic, Berne, IN
The Hope Clinic, Decatur, IN
Women's Care Center, South Bend, IN
Women's Care Center, Plymouth, IN
Women's Care Center, LaPorte, IN
Women's Care Center, Fort Wayne, IN
Women's Care Center, Elkhart, IN
Women's Care Center, Bremen, IN
Women's Care Center, Michigan City, IN
Women's Care Center Inc., Mishawaka, IN

Abortion Recovery Center, Topeka, KS
Advice & Aid Pregnancy Centers, Overland Park, KS
Advice & Aid Pregnancy Centers Inc., Shawnee Mission, KS
Caring Pregnancy Options, Topeka, KS
Open Door Pregnancy Care Center, Hutchinson, KS
Pregnancy Care Center, Augusta, KS
Pregnancy Care Center of Lawrence, Lawrence, KS
Pregnancy Service Center, Salina, KS
Vie Medical Clinic, Pittsburg, KS
Wyandotte Pregnancy Clinic, Kansas City, KS
A Helping Hand Adoption Agency, Lexington, KY
A Woman's Choice Resource Center, Louisville, KY
AA Women's Services, Corbin, KY
Alpha Alternative Pregnancy Care Center, Hopkinsville, KY
Care Net Pregnancy Services of No KY, Cold Springs, KY
Care Net Pregnancy Services of No KY, Florence, KY
Care Net Pregnancy Services of No KY, Williamstown, KY
Care Net Pregnancy Services of Northern Kentucky, Covington, KY
Clarity...Solutions for Women, Elizabethtown, KY
Door of Hope Pregnancy Care Center, Madisonville, KY
Haven of Hope Pregnancy Services, Carrollton, KY
Heart and Soul Life Center, Manchester, KY
Hope Pregnancy Care Center, Morehead, KY
House of Hope Inc., Springfield, KY
Laurel County Life Center, London, KY
Nicole's Place, Louisville, KY
Opportunities for Life, Lexington, KY
Pregnancy Help Center, Richmond, KY
The New Life Center Inc., Bardstown, KY
The Pregnancy Resource Center of Central KY, Danville, KY
Two Hearts Pregnancy Care Centers, Ashland, KY
A Pregnancy Center and Clinic, Lafayette, LA
Access Pregnancy & Referral Centers, Metairie, LA
Community Center for Life, Gretna, LA
Hannah's Plea, A Pregnancy Care Center, Pineville, LA
Hope Restored For Life Inc., Houma, LA
Life Choices Pregnancy Resource Center, Monroe, LA
New Life Counseling, Lake Charles, LA
North Baton Rouge Women's Help Center, Baton Rouge, LA
Northlake Crisis Pregnancy Center, Covington, LA
Sellers Maternity Ministries, Baton Rouge, LA
Woman's New Life Center, Metairie, LA
Women's Life Ministries, Amite, LA
A Woman's Concern, Revere, MA
A Woman's Concern, Dorchester, MA
A Woman's Concern–Cape Cod, Hyannis, MA
A Woman's Concern–North Shore, Beverly, MA
A Woman's Concern–South Coast, Fall River, MA
Alternatives Pregnancy Center, Greenfield, MA
First Concern PRC, Clinton, MA
Pregnancy Care Center, Lawrence, MA
Pregnancy Care Center, Newburyport, MA
Pregnancy Care Center–Seacoast, Amesbury, MA
Pregnancy Care Center of Merrimack Valley, Haverhill, MA
Problem Pregnancy of North Quabbin, Athol, MA
Problem Pregnancy of Worcester Inc., Worcester, MA
Your Life Matters Pregnancy Center, Southbridge, MA
Alpha's Glory Crisis Pregnancy Center, Aberdeen, MD
Bowie Crofton Pregnancy Clinic, Bowie, MD
Catherine Foundation Pregnancy Care Center, Waldorf, MD
Cecil County Pregnancy Center, Elkton, MD
Center for Pregnancy Concerns, Essex, MD
Center for Pregnancy Concerns, Baltimore, MD
Center for Pregnancy Concerns, Dundalk, MD
Centro Tepeyac, Silver Spring WC, Silver Spring, MD
Choices for Life, Easton, MD
Forestville Pregnancy Center, Marlow Heights, MD

Hagerstown Area Pregnancy Center, Hagerstown, MD
Howard County Pregnancy Center, Columbia, MD
Pregnancy Center North, Baltimore, MD
Severna Park Pregnancy Clinic, Severna Park, MD
Shirley Grace Pregnancy Center Inc., Berlin, MD
ABBA–A Women's Resource Center, Portland, ME
Abortion Alternatives Information Inc., Saginaw, MI
Another Way Pregnancy Center, Farmington, MI
Arbor Vitae Women's Center, Ann Arbor, MI
Birth Choice Services, Clarkston, MI
Birthline Pregnancy & Parenting Center, Jackson, MI
Blue Water Pregnancy Care Center, Port Huron, MI
Care Clinic, Marquette, MI
Caring Pregnancy Center, West Branch, MI
Caring Pregnancy Center Iosco, East Tawas, MI
Central Michigan Pregnancy Services, Mt. Pleasant, MI
Crossroads Pregnancy Center, Auburn Hills, MI
Family Life Services of Washtenaw County, Ypsilanti, MI
Heartbeat of Monroe Inc., Monroe, MI
Heartfelt Family Services Inc., Shelby Township, MI
His Love Family Resources, Mio, MI
Life Outreach Center, Houghton, MI
New Beginnings Pregnant Support Services, Ironwood, MI
Oxford Pregnancy Center, Oxford, MI
Pregnancy Aid of Eastern Wayne County, Detroit, MI
Pregnancy Care Center, Traverse City, MI
Pregnancy Help Clinic, Brighton, MI
Pregnancy Resource Center, Grand Rapids, MI
Pregnancy Resource Center, Wyoming, MI
Pregnancy Services of Gratiot County, Alma, MI
The Lennon Pregnancy Center, Dearborn Heights, MI
Walk of Life Pregnancy Services, Iron Mountain, MI
West Shore Pregnancy Care Center, Ludington, MI
Women's Care Center, Niles, MI
Birthline Inc., St. Cloud, MN
Brephos Pregnancy Center, Grand Rapids, MN
Central MN LifeCare Center, Sauk Centre, MN
Chisago Lakes LifeCare Center, Lindstrom, MN
Choices Pregnancy Center, Redwood Falls, MN
First Choice Pregnancy Services, New Ulm, MN
Hastings Total LifeCare Center, Hastings, MN
Health Resources LifeCare Center, Fergus Falls, MN
Highland LifeCare Center, St. Paul, MN
Hope Pregnancy Center, Willmar, MN
Lake Superior LifeCare Center–Duluth, Duluth, MN
Lakes LifeCare Center, Forest Lake, MN
Life Choice Pregnancy Resource Center, Cannon Falls, MN
LifeCare Center East, St. Paul, MN
Minnetonka Life-Care Center, Hopkins, MN
Morris LifeCare Pregnancy Center, Morris, MN
New Beginnings Family Services, Red Wing, MN
New Day Pregnancy Care Center, Little Canada, MN
New Horizons Adoption Agency Inc., Blue Earth, MN
New Life Family Services, Anoka, MN
New Life Family Services, Rochester, MN
New Life Family Services, Minneapolis, MN
New Life Family Services, Richfield, MN
New Life Family Services, St. Paul, MN
North Side Life Care Center, Minneapolis, MN
Northern LifeCare Center, International Falls, MN
Pregnancy Choices LifeCare Center, Apple Valley, MN
Pregnancy LifeCare Center, Hibbing, MN
Pregnancy Options LifeCare Center, Faribault, MN
Pregnancy Resource Center, St. Cloud, MN
Project Life, Stillwater, MN
Thief River Falls LifeCare Center, Thief River Falls, MN
Total Life Care Centers, St. Paul, MN

University LifeCare Center, Minneapolis, MN
Wakota Life-Care Center, West St. Paul, MN
Women's Life Care Center, Little Canada, MN
Women Source, Osseo, MN
Woodbury Life Resource Center, Woodbury, MN
Aaron's House, Harrisonville, MO
Alliance for Life-Missouri, Lee's Summit, MO
Free Women's Center of Pulaski County, Waynesville, MO
Hand 'n Hand Pregnancy Help Center, Barnhart, MO
In HIS Image Ultrasound, Rolla, MO
Jefferson County Pregnancy Care Center, House Springs, MO
Jefferson County Pregnancy Care Center, Crystal City, MO
Life Choice Center for Women, Harrisonville, MO
LifeHouse Crisis Maternity Home, Springfield, MO
Love Basket Inc., Hillsboro, MO
Memphis Area Pregnancy Care Center, Memphis, MO
New Beginnings Women's Center, Warrensburg, MO
North County PRC, Bridgeton, MO
Options Pregnancy Clinic, Branson, MO
Our Lady's Inn, St. Louis, MO
Our Lady's Inn–St. Charles, Defiance, MO
Parkland Pregnancy Resource Center, Park Hills, MO
Pregnancy Care Center, Springfield, MO
Pregnancy Help Center of Central Missouri, Jefferson City, MO
Pregnancy Resource Center of Mountain Grove, Mountain Grove, MO
Pregnancy Resource Center of Rolla, Rolla, MO
Pregnancy Resource Centers–Thrive, St. Louis, MO
Pregnancy Support Center, Lebanon, MO
Rachel House Pregnancy Resource Center, Lee's Summit, MO
Rachel House Pregnancy Resource Center, Blue Springs, MO
Rachel House Pregnancy Resource Center, Kansas City, MO
Riverways Pregnancy Resource Center, Salem, MO
St. Louis City PRC, St. Louis, MO
St. Charles County PRC, St. Peters, MO
The Women's Clinic of Kansas City, Independence, MO
The Women's Clinic of Kansas City, Grandview, MO
Tri County Pregnancy Resource Center, Aurora, MO
CARE Pregnancy Resource Center, Southaven, MS
Center for Pregnancy Choices, Philadelphia, MS
Center for Pregnancy Choices, Meridian, MS
Center for Pregnancy Choices, Vicksburg, MS
Center for Pregnancy Choices–Metro, Jackson, MS
Crisis Pregnancy Center of WBA, Louisville, MS
Center for Pregnancy Choices–Rankin County, Pearl, MS
Pregnancy Resource Center, Wiggins, MS
Women's Resource Center, Gulfport, MS
1st Way Pregnancy Center, Missoula, MT
New Hope Pregnancy Clinic, Butte, MT
St. Catherine Family Health Care Clinic, Belgrade, MT
Sunrise Pregnancy Resource Center, Sidney, MT
Alpha Pregnancy Support Inc., Lexington, NC
Carolina Pregnancy Care Fellowship, Charlotte, NC
Christian Life Home, Raleigh, NC
Crisis Pregnancy Center of Gaston County Inc., Gastonia, NC
Crisis Pregnancy East Gaston, Belmont, NC
Havelock Pregnancy Resource Center, Havelock, NC
HELP Crisis Pregnancy Center, Monroe, NC
In His Hands Pregnancy Support Center, Smithfield, NC
Lois' Lodge, Charlotte, NC
Mooresville Community Pregnancy Center, Mooresville, NC
Pregnancy Resource Center, Charlotte, NC
Room At The Inn Inc., Charlotte, NC
Salem Pregnancy Care Center, Winston-Salem, NC
FirstChoice Clinic, Fargo, ND
FirstChoice Clinic–Lake Region, Devils Lake, ND
FirstChoice Clinic West, Bismarck, ND
Pregnancy Help Center, Park River, ND

Women's Pregnancy Center, Grand Forks, ND
A Woman's Touch, a division of E.P.S., Bellevue, NE
AAA Pregnancy Resource Center, Hastings, NE
ABC Pregnancy Help Center, McCook, NE
Collage Center, Kearney, NE
Essential Pregnancy Services, Omaha, NE
Options For Women, Dover, NH
Choices of the Heart, Turnersville, NJ
Choices of the Heart, Burlington, NJ
Cornerstone Women's Resource Centers, Bridgeton, NJ
Cornerstone Women's Resource Centers, Salem, NJ
Friendship Center for New Beginnings, Flemington, NJ
Gateway Pregnancy Center, Irvington, NJ
Gateway Pregnancy Center, Elizabeth, NJ
Gateway Pregnancy Center, Plainfield, NJ
Life Choices Resource Center, Metuchen, NJ
Lighthouse Pregnancy Resource Center, Hackensack, NJ
Lighthouse Pregnancy Resource Center, Hawthorne, NJ
Pregnancy Aid & Information Center Inc., Raritan, NJ
Animas Pregnancy Center, Farmington, NM
Life Choice Center, Clovis, NM
New Life Pregnancy Center, Taos, NM
Turning Point of Las Cruces Inc., Las Cruces, NM
Culture of Life Coalition, Reno Tahoe, Reno, NV
First Choice Pregnancy Services, Las Vegas, NV
AAA Pregnancy Options, Hempstead, NY
AAA Pregnancy Options, Deer Park, NY
Alight Care Center, Troy, NY
Alight Care Center, Margaretville, NY
Alight Pregnancy Center Inc., Hudson, NY
All Med Clinic, Bronx, NY
Choose Life/Women's Services, Jamestown, NY
Expectant Mother Care Pregnancy Center, Yonkers, NY
Expectant Mother Care Pregnancy Center, Brooklyn, NY
Expectant Mother Care Pregnancy Center, New York, NY
Expectant Mother Care Pregnancy Center, Bronx, NY
Expectant Mother Care Pregnancy Center, Corona, NY
Expectant Mother Care Pregnancy Center, Hollis, NY
Expectant Mother Care Pregnancy Center, Richmond Hill, NY
Expectant Mother Care Pregnancy Center, Brooklyn, NY
Life Center of Long Island, Massapequa, NY
Lockport Care Net Pregnancy Center, Lockport, NY
Midtown Pregnancy Support Center, New York, NY
New Hope Family Services, Syracuse, NY
Pregnancy Help Inc., New York, NY
Pregnancy Resource Services, Staten Island, NY
Premium Healthcare Clinic, New York, NY
Summit Life Outreach Center Inc., Niagara Falls, NY
The Care Center, Islandia, NY
Tri-County Crisis Pregnancy Center, Gowanda, NY
A Caring Place Pregnancy Help Center, Cincinnati, OH
Adams County Pregnancy Resource Center, West Union, OH
AIM Women's Center & Clinic, Steubenville, OH
Alternaterm Pregnancy Services, Cleveland Heights, OH
Ashland Care Center Inc., Ashland, OH
Bethel Ministries–Voice of Hope PC, Upper Sandusky, OH
Bowling Green Pregnancy Center, Bowling Green, OH
Cleveland Pregnancy Center, Cleveland, OH
Cleveland Pregnancy Center, Berea, OH
Clinton County Women's Center, Wilmington, OH
Community Pregnancy Center, Barberton, OH
Community Pregnancy Centers, Defiance, OH
Community Pregnancy Centers, Wauseon, OH
Community Pregnancy Centers of NW Ohio, Bryan, OH
Cornerstone Among Women, Rocky River, OH
Cornerstone Among Women, Elyria, OH
Darlene Bishop Home for Life Inc., Monroe, OH

Elizabeth's Hope Pregnancy Resources, Circleville, OH
Elizabeth's Hope Pregnancy Resources, Chillicothe, OH
Elizabeth's Hope Pregnancy Resources, Waverly, OH
Elizabeth's Hope Pregnancy Resources, Jackson, OH
Elizabeth's New Life Center, Dayton, OH
Fairborn Women's Network, Fairborn, OH
Family Life Center of Auglaize County, St. Marys, OH
FYI's Women's Network, New Carlisle, OH
Heartbeat Family Center Inc., Zanesville, OH
Heartbeat of Columbiana County Inc., East Liverpool, OH
Heartbeat of Fremont, Fremont, OH
Heartbeat of Hardin County, Kenton, OH
Heartbeat of Morrow County Inc., Mt. Gilead, OH
Heartbeat of Ottawa County, Port Clinton, OH
Heartbeat of Sandusky, Sandusky, OH
Heartbeat of Toledo Inc., Toledo, OH
Heartbeat Pregnancy Center, Port Clinton, OH
Heartbeats of Licking County, Newark, OH
L.I.F.E. Pregnancy Center, Washington Court House, OH
Lifepointe Family Center, London, OH
Miami Valley Women's Center, Dayton, OH
Miami Valley Women's Center, Xenia, OH
Miami Valley Women's Center, Huber Heights, OH
Navarre Park–East Toledo Family Center, Toledo, OH
Pregnancy Care of Summit County, Akron, OH
Pregnancy Center East, Cincinnati, OH
Pregnancy Center of Greater Toledo, Toledo, OH
Pregnancy Center of Kent, Kent, OH
Pregnancy Center West Inc., Cincinnati, OH
Pregnancy Decision Health Centers, Columbus, OH
Pregnancy Decision Health Centers, Lancaster, OH
Pregnancy Help Center, Youngstown, OH
Pregnancy Life Center, Van Wert, OH
Pregnancy Resource Center, Mt. Orab, OH
Pregnancy Resource Center, Georgetown, OH
Pregnancy Support Center, Canton, OH
Pregnancy Support Center, Massillon, OH
Pregnancy Care of Cincinnati, Cincinnati, OH
PSC of Stark County, Canton, OH
Reach Out Pregnancy Center, Harrison, OH
Relationships Under Construction, Delaware, OH
Richland Pregnancy Services, Mansfield, OH
Southern Ohio Pregnancy Center, Hillsboro, OH
Spirit of Faith Adoptions, Sylvania, OH
Springfield Women's Network, Springfield, OH
The CORE Center, Delaware, OH
The Women's Clinic of Columbus, Columbus, OH
Two Hearts of Lawrence County, Coal Grove, OH
Vineyard Columbus, Westerville, OH
Voice of Hope Pregnancy Center, Bucyrus, OH
Voice of Hope Pregnancy Center, Marion, OH
Women's Care Center, Columbus, OH
Women's Center–East, Dayton, OH
Women's Center–Kettering, Dayton, OH
Women's Center–Lebanon, Lebanon, OH
Women's Center–Sidney, Sidney, OH
Abundant Blessings Center, Grove, OK
Lighthouse Pregnancy Center, Jay, OK
Mend Medical Clinic/PRC, Tulsa, OK
Pregnancy Resource Center of Southern Oklahoma, Ardmore, OK
Stillwater Life Services Inc., Stillwater, OK
Next Step Pregnancy Information Center, La Grande, OR
Pregnancy Alternatives Center, Lebanon, OR
Pregnancy Center of the Illinois Valley, Cave Junction, OR
A Woman's Concern Inc., Lancaster, PA
ABC Pregnancy Center, Franklin, PA
Blessed Margaret Home, Bensalem, PA

Care Net of Scranton, Scranton, PA
Care Net Pregnancy Center of NEPA, Montrose, PA
Columbia Pregnancy Center, Columbia, PA
Crisis Pregnancy Center of Greene County, Waynesburg, PA
Crossroads Pregnancy Center, Lewistown, PA
Crossroads Pregnancy Center, Mt. Union, PA
Crossroads Pregnancy Center, Huntingdon, PA
Crossroads Pregnancy Center, Mifflin, PA
Ephrata Pregnancy Center, Ephrata, PA
Lancaster Pregnancy Clinic, Lancaster, PA
Lebanon Pregnancy Clinic, Lebanon, PA
Lifeline of Berks County, West Reading, PA
Lifeline Pregnancy Care Center, Millersburg, PA
Life-Way Pregnancy Center, Latrobe, PA
Life-Way Pregnancy Clinic, Indiana, PA
Loving and Caring Inc., Lancaster, PA
Mary's Shelter, Reading, PA
Morning Star Pregnancy Services, Harrisburg, PA
Morning Star Pregnancy Services, Middletown, PA
Morning Star Pregnancy Services, New Cumberland, PA
My Choice Medical Clinic, Kittanning, PA
Pregnancy Care Center, Coal Township, PA
Pregnancy Resource Clinic of N Penn, Lansdale, PA
Pregnancy Resource Center, New Castle, PA
Pregnancy Services of Western PA, Sharon, PA
Pregnancy Support Center of Warren County, Warren, PA
Slate Belt Pregnancy Support Services Inc., Bangor, PA
Slippery Rock Pregnancy Center, Slippery Rock, PA
Susquehanna Valley Pregnancy Services, Lebanon, PA
Tender Care Pregnancy Consultation Services, Hanover, PA
Tender Care Pregnancy Consultation Services, Gettysburg, PA
Tri-City Life Center, Lower Burrell, PA
Tri-State Pregnancy Center, Matamoras, PA
Twin Tiers Pregnancy Care Center, Bradford, PA
Women's Care Center, Erie, PA
Women's Care Center, Union City, PA
CAM–San Juan, PR, Guaynabo, PR
CareNet Pregnancy Center of RI, Providence, RI
Mother of Life Center, Providence, RI
Mother of Life Center, Westerly, RI
Beaufort Women's Center, Beaufort, SC
Carolina Family Planning Centers, Hartsville, SC
Carolina Family Planning Centers, Darlington, SC
Christian Family Services, Rock Hill, SC
Foothills Pregnancy Care Center, Seneca, SC
Lowcountry Crisis Pregnancy Center, Charleston, SC
Lowcountry Pregnancy Center, N Charleston, SC
Nightlight Christian Adoptions, Greenville, SC
Options Medical Clinic, Gaffney, SC
Pregnancy Center and Clinic, Hilton Head, SC
Alpha Center, Sioux Falls, SD
Mitchell Area Prolife Coalition, Mitchell, SD
New Horizons Adoption Agency Inc., Sioux Falls, SD
Choices Pregnancy Resource Center, Chattanooga, TN
Choices Resource Center, Oak Ridge, TN
Grace Pregnancy Resource Center, Nashville, TN
Heartbeat Haven Pregnancy Resource Center, Lafayette, TN
Life Choices of Memphis, Memphis, TN
Life Choices of Memphis Inc., Memphis, TN
Pregnancy Help Center, Knoxville, TN
Pregnancy Help Center, Chattanooga, TN
Pregnancy Help Center, La Follette, TN
Pregnancy Help Center, Carthage, TN
Pregnancy Resource Center, Maryville, TN
Women's Care Center of Sevier County Inc., Sevierville, TN
Adoption Angels, San Antonio, TX
Adoption Priorities Inc., San Antonio, TX

Anchor Point, League City, TX
Arlington Pregnancy Center–SE, Arlington, TX
Arlington Pregnancy Center–SW, Arlington, TX
Arlington-Mansfield Pregnancy Centers, Arlington, TX
Austin LifeCare, Austin, TX
Birth Choice of Dallas, Dallas, TX
Burleson Pregnancy Aid Center, Burleson, TX
Dallas Pregnancy Resource Center, Dallas, TX
Downtown Pregnancy Center, Dallas, TX
Downtown Pregnancy Help Center, Houston, TX
Eastland County Open Door, Cisco, TX
Fannin Pregnancy Care Center, Bonham, TX
Fifth Ward Pregnancy Help Center, Houston, TX
First Choice Pregnancy Resource Center, Texarkana, TX
Fort Worth Pregnancy Center, Fort Worth, TX
Generations Adoptions, Waco, TX
Heartbeat Pregnancy Center, Nacogdoches, TX
Heartline Women's Clinic, Lubbock, TX
Heartworks Pregnancy Resource Center, Longview, TX
Highland Lakes Pregnancy Resource Center, Kingsland, TX
Hope Connections PRC, Leander, TX
Hope Resource Center of McKinney, McKinney, TX
House of Hope, El Paso, TX
Life Talk Resource Center, Frisco, TX
Living Alternatives of Palestine, Palestine, TX
McAllen Pregnancy Center, McAllen, TX
Mid Cities Pregnancy Center, North Richland Hills, TX
Mid Cities Pregnancy Center, Irving, TX
New Life Pregnancy Center, Houston, TX
New Life Pregnancy Center, Magnolia, TX
Paris Pregnancy Care Center, Paris, TX
Paris Pregnancy Care Center–Athens, Athens, TX
Pflugerville Pregnancy Resource Center, Pflugerville, TX
Pregnancy Assistance Center North, The Woodlands, TX
Pregnancy Assistance Center North, Conroe, TX
Pregnancy Care Center of Texoma, Sherman, TX
Pregnancy Care Center–Huntsville, Huntsville, TX
Pregnancy Help Center, Vernon, TX
Pregnancy Help Center, Lake Jackson, TX
Pregnancy Help Center, Wichita Falls, TX
Pregnancy Help Center of West Houston, Katy, TX
Pregnancy Resource Center, Rockwall, TX
Pregnancy Resource Center, Mesquite, TX
Pregnancy Resource Center of Ft. Bend County, Rosenberg, TX
Pregnancy Resource Center of Ft. Bend County, Sugar Land, TX
Pregnancy Resource Center-Grand Prairie, Grand Prairie, TX
Pregnancy Resources of Abilene, Abilene, TX
Prestonwood Pregnancy Center, Dallas, TX
Raffa Clinic, Greenville, TX
Raffa Clinic, Commerce, TX
Sound Options Pregnancy Services, Duncanville, TX
South Austin Pregnancy Resource Center, Austin, TX
South Texas Pregnancy Care Center, Seguin, TX
Still Waters, Kaufman, TX
The Haven, Clyde, TX
The John Paul II Life Center, Austin, TX
The Life Center, Midland, TX
The Life Center, Andrews, TX
The Pregnancy Resource Center, Kerrville, TX
White Rose Women's Center, Dallas, TX
Wise Choices Pregnancy Resource Center, Decatur, TX
Woman to Woman Pregnancy Resource Center, Denton, TX
Women's Choice Resource Center, Fort Worth, TX
Women's Resource Center of East Texas, Forney, TX
WRC Pregnancy Center of Ellis County, Ennis, TX
WRC Pregnancy Center of Ellis County, Waxahachie, TX
1st Choice Women's Health Center, Lansdowne, VA

Alexandria Pregnancy Help Center, Alexandria, VA
Assist Pregnancy Center, Annandale, VA
Bedford Pregnancy Center, Bedford, VA
Blue Ridge Pregnancy Center, Lynchburg, VA
Blue Ridge Women's Center, Roanoke, VA
Care Net Pregnancy Resource Centers, Warrenton, VA
Care Net Pregnancy Resource Centers, Woodbridge, VA
Care Net Pregnancy Resource Centers, Manassas, VA
Crisis Pregnancy Center of Tidewater, Norfolk, VA
Fairfax Pregnancy Help Center, Fairfax, VA
Front Royal Pregnancy Center, Front Royal, VA
Harrisonburg Pregnancy Center, Harrisonburg, VA
Lady Care Inc., Chesapeake, VA
LifeChoices Resource Center, Fairfax, VA
Little Life Pregnancy Center, Danville, VA
Mary's Shelter Inc., Fredericksburg, VA
Pregnancy Resource Center of Metro Richmond, Richmond, VA
Pregnancy Resource Center of the NRV, Blacksburg, VA
The Keim Center of Norfolk, Norfolk, VA
The Keim Center of Portsmouth, Portsmouth, VA
The Keim Center of Suffolk, Suffolk, VA
The Keim Center of Virginia Beach, Virginia Beach, VA
Care Center Family Life and Pregnancy Resource Center, Centralia, WA
Care Net Pregnancy & Family Services, Puyallup, WA
Care Net Pregnancy & Family Services, Federal Way, WA
Care Net Pregnancy & Family Services, Tacoma, WA
Care Net Pregnancy & Family Services, Kenmore, WA
Care Net Pregnancy & Family Services, Gig Harbor, WA
Care Net Pregnancy & Family Services, Lakewood, WA
i-CHOICE/Life Services Cheney Center, Cheney, WA
Life Services of Spokane, Spokane, WA
N.E.W. Family Life Services, Colville, WA
Next Step Pregnancy Services, Lynnwood, WA
Pregnancy Care Clinic, Oak Harbor, WA
Pregnancy Support Service of Ephrata, Ephrata, WA
South Whidbey Clinic, Langley, WA
Whatcom County Pregnancy Clinic, Bellingham, WA
Abiding Care Pregnancy Resource Center, Medford, WI
Alpha Center, Racine, WI
Bella Medical Clinic, Oshkosh, WI
Hartford Pregnancy Help Center, Hartford, WI
Lake Superior LifeCare Center–Superior, Superior, WI
Pregnancy Helpline, Madison, WI
Pregnancy Helpline LifeCare Center, River Falls, WI
Pregnancy Helpline of Janesville Inc., Janesville, WI
Pregnancy Helpline of Walworth County, Elkhorn, WI
Pregnancy Resource Center, Portage, WI
Stateline Pregnancy Clinic, Beloit, WI
The Crossing of Manitowoc County Inc., Manitowoc, WI
Tri-County LifeCare Center, Osceola, WI
Waupaca Pregnancy Information Center, Waupaca, WI
WomanKind Medical Clinic, Appleton, WI
Women's Care Center, Milwaukee, WI
Women's Support Centers, Milwaukee, WI
Care Pregnancy Center, Shepherdstown, WV
Care Pregnancy Center of the Eastern Panhandle, Martinsburg, WV
Central WV Center for Pregnancy Care, Thomas, WV
Central WV Center for Pregnancy Care, Buckhannon, WV
Central WV Center for Pregnancy Care, Parsons, WV
My Father's House Inc., Martinsburg, WV
Pregnancy Resource Center of Marion County, Fairmont, WV
TLC Pregnancy Center of Ritchie County, Ellenboro, WV
Woman's Choice PRC, Charleston, WV
Care Net Pregnancy & Resource Clinic, Casper, WY
Heart to Heart, Laramie, WY
Legacy Pregnancy Resource Center, Sheridan, WY
Serenity Pregnancy Resource Center, Cody, WY

Women's Resource Center of NE WY, Gillette, WY
Brooks Pregnancy Care Centre, Brooks, AB, Canada
Calgary Pregnancy Care Centre, Calgary, AB, Canada
CAPSS Canada National Office, Red Deer, AB, Canada
Central Alberta PCC, Red Deer, AB, Canada
Christian Adoption Services, Calgary, AB, Canada
Cochrane Pregnancy Care Center, Cochrane, AB, Canada
High Level Women's Support Center, High Level, AB, Canada
Pregnancy Care Centre, Edmonton, AB, Canada
West Yellowhead Pregnancy Care Centre, Hinton, AB, Canada
Christian Advocacy Society, Burnaby, BC, Canada
Comox Valley Pregnancy Care Centre, Courtenay, BC, Canada
CPC of Burnaby & New Westminster, Burnaby, BC, Canada
Crisis Pregnancy Centre of Nanaimo Society, Nanaimo, BC, Canada
Crisis Pregnancy Centre of Vancouver, Vancouver, BC, Canada
Fraser Valley Crisis Pregnancy Society, Aldergrove, BC, Canada
Nelson Crisis Pregnancy Centre, Nelson, BC, Canada
North Peace Pregnancy Care Centre Society, Fort St. John, BC, Canada
Okanagan Valley Pregnancy Care Centre, Kelowna, BC, Canada
Options Pregnancy Centre, Victoria, BC, Canada
Post Abortion Community Services, Burnaby, BC, Canada
Pregnancy Care Centre Society, Kamloops, BC, Canada
Pregnancy Concerns, Coquitlam, BC, Canada
Prince George Crisis Pregnancy Centre, Prince George, BC, Canada
Pro Life BC, Abbotsford, BC, Canada
South Fraser Pregnancy Options Society, Surrey, BC, Canada
WomanCare Pregnancy Centre, Maple Ridge, BC, Canada
Crisis Pregnancy Centre of Westman Inc., Brandon, MB, Canada
Grace Haven Pregnancy Crisis Centre, Steinbach, MB, Canada
Northern Pregnancy Care Centre Inc., Flin Flon, MB, Canada
Pembina Valley Pregnancy Care Centre, Winkler, MB, Canada
The Family Support Centre of Winnipeg, Winnipeg, MB, Canada
Fundy Crisis Pregnancy Centre, St. John, NB, Canada
Pregnancy Resource Centre of Moncton, Moncton, NB, Canada
Sussex and Area Crisis Pregnancy Centre, Sussex, NB, Canada
Metro Pregnancy and Family Support Centre, Halifax, NS, Canada
The Valley Care Pregnancy Centre, Kentville, NS, Canada
Tri-County Pregnancy Care Centre, Yarmouth, NS, Canada
Tri-County Pregnancy Care Centre, Barrington Passage, NS, Canada
Algoma Crisis Pregnancy Centre, Sault Ste. Marie, ON, Canada
Anchor of Hope Crisis Pregnancy Centre, Madoc, ON, Canada
Bancroft Pregnancy Care Centre, Bancroft, ON, Canada
Barrie Pregnancy Resource Centre, Barrie, ON, Canada
Beginnings Counseling/Adoption Services, Hamilton, ON, Canada
Beginnings Family Services, Guelph, ON, Canada
Beginnings Pregnancy Care Centre, Cobourg, ON, Canada
Belleville Pregnancy and Family Care Centre, Belleville, ON, Canada
Brampton Life Centre, Brampton, ON, Canada
Caledonia Centre, Caledonia, ON, Canada
Cambridge Pregnancy Resource Centre, Cambridge, ON, Canada
Elisha House Pregnancy and Family Support Centre, Welland, ON, Canada
First Place Pregnancy Centre, Ottawa, ON, Canada
Haldiman Pregnancy Care Centre, Dunnville, ON, Canada
Hannah House, Niagara Falls, ON, Canada
Haven on the Queensway, Toronto, ON, Canada
Highlands Community Pregnancy Care Centre, Haliburton, ON, Canada
Huronia Crisis Pregnancy Centre, Midland, ON, Canada
Island Pregnancy Care and Support Services, Charlottetown, ON, Canada
K–W Pregnancy Resource Centre, Waterloo, ON, Canada
Kingston Crisis Pregnancy Centre, Kingston, ON, Canada
Lambton Crisis Pregnancy Centre, Sarnia, ON, Canada
Lindsay Crisis Pregnancy Centre, Lindsay, ON, Canada
London Crisis Pregnancy Centre, London, ON, Canada
Markham/Stouffville Crisis Pregnancy Centre, Markham, ON, Canada
Mississauga Life Centre, Mississauga, ON, Canada
Nigeria Life League, Toronto, ON, Canada
Norfolk Pregnancy Centre, Simcoe, ON, Canada
North Shore Pregnancy Care Center, Blind River, ON, Canada
North York Pregnancy Care Centre, Toronto, ON, Canada
Orillia Pregnancy Resource Centre, Orillia, ON, Canada
Owen Sound Crisis Pregnancy Centre, Owen Sound, ON, Canada
Peterborough Pregnancy Support Services, Peterborough, ON, Canada
Pregnancy & Resource Centre, Brantford, ON, Canada
Pregnancy Care Centre, Toronto, ON, Canada
Pregnancy Care Centre of Sudbury, Sudbury, ON, Canada
Pregnancy Support Services of Upper Ottawa Valley, Pembroke, ON, Canada
Prince Edward Pregnancy and Family Care Centre, Picton, ON, Canada
Sara's Place Maternity Home, Stratford, ON, Canada
South Niagara Life Centre, Fort Erie, ON, Canada
Stratford House of Blessing, Stratford, ON, Canada
Sunparlour Pregnancy Resource Centre, Windsor, ON, Canada
Sunparlour Pregnancy Resource Centre, Leamington, ON, Canada
TLC Pregnancy Centre, Newmarket, ON, Canada
Uxbridge Pregnancy Centre, Uxbridge, ON, Canada
Centre D'aide Oasis Care Centre, Verdun, QC, Canada
Montreal Youth Unlimited, Chateauguay, QC, Canada
Options Grossesse, Quebec City, QC, Canada
Options Pregnancy Center, Resources and Lifestyle Coaching, Regina, SK, Canada
Real Choices for Women and Families: Family Life Support, Saskatoon, SK, Canada
Ame La Merced/CAM, Buenos Aires, Argentina
CAM–Garin, Provincia de Buenos Aires, Argentina
CAM–Lujan, Buenos Aires, Argentina
Pro familia/CAM, Buenos Aires, Argentina
VITAM/CAM–Pilar, Buenos Aires, Argentina
Gravida, Centro de Asistencia, San Pedro, Argentina
VITAM/CAM, Mendoza, Argentina
Word of Life Pregnancy Care Center, Yerevan, Armenia
Pregnancy Support Service (ACT), Civic Square, Australia
CatholicCare Pregnancy Counselling, Bankstown, Australia
Diamond Pregnancy Support Inc., Baulkham Hills, BC, Australia
Doonside/Mt. Druitt PHC, Doonside, Australia
Manning Pregnancy Support Inc., Taree, Australia
Newcastle Pregnancy Help Service, The Junction, Australia
Pregnancy Care Coffs Harbour, Coffs Harbour, Australia
Pregnancy Help Australia Limited, Toormina, Australia
Pregnancy Help Campbelltown, Liverpool BC, Australia
Pregnancy Help Center Manly/Warringah, Brookvale, Australia
Pregnancy Help Midcoast, West Kempsey, Australia
Pregnancy Help Sydney, Liverpool BC, Australia
Pregnancy Support Line, Beacon Hill, Australia
Pregnancy Support Parramatta, Baulkham Hills, Australia
Pregnancy & Family Support Gold Coast, Burleigh Heads, Australia
Pregnancy Help Mackay, Mackay, Australia
Priceless Life Centre, Alderly, Australia
Birthline Pregnancy Support Inc., Kensington Gardens, Australia
Genesis Pregnancy Support Inc., Plympton, Australia
Pregnancy Counselling & Support Tas, Hobart, Australia
Your Choice, New Town, Australia
Billings Ovulation Method, East Burwood, Australia
Pregnancy Help Geelong Inc., Geelong, Australia
Real Choices Australia, Wodonga, Australia
Crisis Pregnancy Care, Pinjarra, Australia
Pregnancy Help Bunbury, Bunbury, Australia
Pregnancy Problem House, Northlands, Australia
Elohim Heartbeat, Nassau, New Providence, Bahamas
Gomel "Protection of Babies," Gomel, Belarus
Seed of Life–CAM–Belize, Belize
SEED of Life Pregnancy Resource Center, Benque Viejo del Carmen, Cayo, Belize

CAM–Cochabamba, Cochabamba, Bolivia
CAM–La Paz, La Paz, Bolivia
Red Vida de Esperanza, Cochabamba, Casilla, Bolivia
CERVI, Sao Paulo, Brazil
Women Pro-Life Info Center, Sofia, Bulgaria
Life Care Network, Bamenda, Cameroon
Lumen Dei–Santiago, Santiago, Chile
Movimiento Anonimo por la Vida, Santiago, Chile
CAM–Zipaquira, Zipaquira, Cundinamarca, Colombia
CAM–Palmira Valle, Palmira Valle, Colombia
CAM–San Jose Cucuta, San Jose de Cucuta, Colombia
CAM–San Jose Guaviare, San Jose de Guaviare, Colombia
CAM–Villavicencio, Villavicencio, Colombia
CEDIME, San Jose, Colombia
Centro de Apoyo a la Mujer–CAM, Bogota, Colombia
Centro Internacional para Mujeres, Barranquilla, Atlantico, Colombia
Lumen Dei–CAM, Bogota, Colombia
Lumen Dei/Cali–CAM, Cali, Colombia
Lumen Dei/Medellin–CAM, Medellin, Colombia
Provida Digna, Cali, Colombia
Refugio de Maria, Medellin, Colombia
Mami–CAM, Ibague, Colombia
CAM–La Habana, La Habana, Cuba
Hjerte for Liv (Heart for Life), Aalborg, Denmark
CAM–Ambato, Ambato, Ecuador
CAM–Cuenca, Cuenca, Ecuador
CAM–Guayaquil, Guayaquil, Ecuador
CAM–Quito/Centro, Quito/Centro, Ecuador
CAM–Quito/Matriz, Quito/Matriz, Ecuador
FLEXIPLAST, Quito, Ecuador
Yo Mujer–CAM, Quito, Ecuador
Fundacion Si a la Vida–CAM, Santa Tecla, La Libertad, El Salvador
Valgus Linnas, Tartu, Estonia
Ethiopian Women/Children Life Centre, Addis Ababa, Ethiopia
Kaiserslautern Crisis Pregnancy Center, Kaiserslautern-Einsiedlerhof,
    Germany
Destiny Changers International, Accra, Ghana
Fordjour's Counseling Center, Mamprobi-Accra, Ghana
Heartbeat Ghana Ministries, Accra, Ghana
International Hope Centre for Women, Accra, Ghana
Life Center of Ghana, Adum Kumasi, Ghana
Life International Center of Ghana, Adum Kumasi, Ghana
POWERAID, Accra, Ghana
Hope for Life, Neo Faliro Pireaus, Greece
APROVI–CAM, Guatemala, Guatemala
Si a la Vida–CAM, Guatemala, Guatemala
House of Hope, Sayaxche, Guatemala
Mercy & Grace Charitable Trust, Krishna District, India
Care & Share Ministry, Chennai, India
Christo Development Trust, Udumalpet, India
Jakarta Pregnancy Center, Jakarta Sultan, Indonesia
Ask Majella Pregnancy Advisory Services, Limerick, Ireland
Pro Life–Human Life, Waterford, Ireland
A Future And A Hope, Yerushalayim, Israel
Be'ad Chaim Association, Jerusalem, Israel
Crisis Pregnancy Ministries (YFC), Nairobi, Kenya
Nyamira Adventist Medical Centre, Nyamira, Nyanza, Kenya
Protecting Life Movement, Nairobi, Kenya
Te Mak Ministries, Kisumu, Kenya
Wholistic Caring & Counseling Center, Ruiru, Kenya
Options, Ladybrand, Lesotho
Maoni Orphanage, Blantyre, Malawi
CAM–Distrito Federal, Distrito Federal, Mexico
RED Latinoamericana de CAMs, Distrito Federal, Mexico
House of Grace PCC, Rehoboth, Namibia
Voice of Fetus Nepal, Kathmandu, Nepal
LIfe Center Victoria House, Zwolle, Netherlands

9 Months Plus Charitable Trust, Christchurch, New Zealand
The House of Grace Trust Inc., Wellington, New Zealand
CAM–Managua, Managua, Nicaragua
Abandoned Children/Women/Orphans, Jos, Nigeria
Incredible Doors, Ilorin, Nigeria
Life Helpers Initiative, Sokoto, Nigeria
Project for Human Development, Surulere, Nigeria
Pro-life Evangel, Jos, Nigeria
Lumen Dei/Arequipa–CAM, Arequipa, Peru
Movimiento Sadalicio–CAM, Arequipa, Peru
Lumen Dei /Cusco–CAM, Cusco, Peru
CEPROFARENA–CAM, Lima, Peru
Lumen Dei/Lima–CAM, Lima, Peru
Pregnancy Support Services of Asia, EDSA, Guadalupe, Makati City,
    Philippines
Ministerio Pro-vida Raquel, San Juan, Puerto Rico
Choose Life Center, Novi Sad, Vojvodina, Serbia
Abba Pregnancy Crisis Centre, Gonubie, South Africa
Alternatives Pregnancy Crisis Centre, Humewood, South Africa
New Life Crisis Pregnancy Centre, Mosel, South Africa
PLIGHT Crisis Pregnancy Centre, Port Alfred, South Africa
Springtime Crisis Pregnancy Center, Grahamstown, South Africa
Zoe Life Centre, Welkom, South Africa
Bethany Pregnancy Crisis Centre, Lyttleton, South Africa
Born 2 Care–Heidelberg, Heidelberg, South Africa
Destiny Pregnancy Crisis Centre, Freemanville, Klerksdorp, South
    Africa
Galgotha Ministries, Vosloorus, South Africa
Hope/Themba Crisis Pregnancy Centre, Petersfield, South Africa
Neo Birth Pregnancy Crisis Centre, Hatfield, South Africa
Neobirth–Rustenburg, Rustenburg, South Africa
Tshepo Woman Help Centre, Boksburg, South Africa
Zoe Pregnancy Crisis Centre, Rynfield, Benoni, South Africa
Africa Cares for Life, Seadoone, South Africa
Angels of Mercy, Montclair, South Africa
KwaZulu Department of Health, Eshowe, South Africa
New Hope Ministries, Pinetown, South Africa
Pregnancy Resource Centre, Doonside, South Africa
Turning Point Pregnancy Crisis Centre, Uvongo, South Africa
Options CPC (Youth for Christ), Knysna, South Africa
Options CPC (Youth for Christ), George, South Africa
Anchor of Hope, Viliersdorp, South Africa
Help Pregnancy Crisis Centre, Worcester, South Africa
New Life Centre, Bellville, South Africa
Options Care Centre–Montague, Montague Gardens, South Africa
Pregnancy Help Centre, Tokai, South Africa
Seasons Pregnancy Centre, Stellenbosch, South Africa
Adoptions 4 Ever, Phalaborwa, South Africa
Born 2 Care, Delmas, South Africa
Centre of Hope Clinic, Durban, South Africa
Jogebed Pregnancy Crisis Centre, Upington, South Africa
Kwamashu Christian Centre, Marbleray, South Africa
Life Link Pregnancy Care Centre, Aston Manor, South Africa
Fundacion Madrina, Madrid, Spain
Ray of Hope CPC, Tainan, Taiwan
The Elpis Centre, Debe, Trinidad and Tobago
Human Life International Uganda, Kampala, Uganda
Crisis Pregnancy Counseling Centre, Kampala City, Uganda
The Comforter's Centre, Kampala, Uganda
Viva Network–CRANE, Kampala, Uganda
Advocates For Life International, Kitwe, Zambia
Silent Voices, Kitwe, Zambia

Appendix VI: Our Commitment of Care and Competence

1. Clients are served without regard to age, race, income, nationality, religious affiliation, disability, or other arbitrary circumstances.
2. Clients are treated with kindness, compassion, and in a caring manner.
3. Clients always receive honest and open answers.
4. Client pregnancy tests are distributed and administered in accordance with all applicable laws.
5. Client information is held in strict and absolute confidence. Releases and permissions are obtained appropriately. Client information is only disclosed as required by law and when necessary to protect the client or others against imminent harm.
6. Clients receive accurate information about pregnancy, fetal development, lifestyle issues, and related concerns.
7. We do not offer, recommend, or refer for abortions or abortifacients, but are committed to offering accurate information about abortion procedures and risks.
8. All of our advertising and communication are truthful and honest and accurately describe the services we offer.
9. We provide a safe environment by screening all volunteers and staff interacting with clients.
10. We are governed by a board of directors and operate in accordance with our articles of incorporation, bylaws, and stated purpose and mission.
11. We comply with applicable legal and regulatory requirements regarding employment, fundraising, financial management, taxation, and public disclosure, including the filing of all applicable government reports in a timely manner.
12. Medical services are provided in accordance with all applicable laws and in accordance with pertinent medical standards, under the supervision and direction of a licensed physician.
13. All of our staff, board members, and volunteers receive appropriate training to uphold these standards.

About the Author

Margaret H. (Peggy) Hartshorn, Ph.D., became involved in the pro-life movement soon after the Supreme Court decision *Roe v. Wade* on January 22, 1973.

Peggy and her husband joined the local Right to Life group, and they began housing pregnant women in their home in 1975. They opened Pregnancy Decision Health Centers in Columbus, Ohio, on January 22, 1981, where Peggy served as chairman of the board for more than twenty years. Under her leadership, PDHC became one of the first pregnancy centers to offer ultrasound services. It grew to five locations, serving more than 15,000 hotline and office clients annually.

In 1993, Peggy resigned from her job as a professor of English at Franklin University in Columbus, Ohio, to become the first full-time president of Heartbeat International. Under her leadership, Heartbeat has grown from a network of 250 affiliated pregnancy help centers to the most expansive network of pregnancy help ministries in the world, about 1,200 pregnancy help centers, medical clinics, maternity homes, nonprofit adoption agencies, and abortion recovery programs in more than fifty countries.

In 2008 in Washington, D.C., the Gerard Health Foundation recognized Peggy with one of the inaugural Life Prize awards. In 2007, she received the Cardinal John J. O'Connor Pro-Life award from Legatus International. She has also received the Patrick Cardinal O'Boyle Award from the Fellowship of Catholic Scholars, the J.C. Penney Golden Rule Award, the Sanctity of Human Life Award from Care Net, and the Founder's Award from the Christ Child Society. The Diocese of Columbus, Ohio, named her Catholic Woman of the Year in 2004.

Peggy has been married to Michael Hartshorn for forty-two years. They have two adopted children, now married, and five grandchildren.